TIME MANAGEMENT FOR ADULTS WITH ADHD

FROM OVERWHELM TO ORDER: HOW TO TAKE CONTROL OF YOUR TIME AND THRIVE WITH ADHD

NOELLE WALKER

TABLE OF CONTENTS

Authors Note   7
Introduction   11

1. UNDERSTANDING ADHD AND TIME
MANAGEMENT   15
Decoding Time Blindness in ADHD   16
The Relationship Between Executive Dysfunction
and Procrastination   17
Overcoming Hyperfocus: Balancing Intense
Concentration With Time Awareness   19
Emotional Regulation and Its Role in Time
Management   21
ADHD and Impulsivity: Strategies for Controlling
Spur-Of-The-Moment Decisions   23

2. CUSTOM TOOLS AND TECHNIQUES FOR
EVERYDAY PRODUCTIVITY   27
Designing Your ADHD-Friendly Daily Planner   27
Time Blindness Techniques for the ADHD Mind   30
Setting up Effective Reminders and Alarms   33
The Role of Visual Aids in Managing Time   35
Building Routine With ADHD: A Step-By-Step
Guide   38

3. TACKLING COMMON ADHD TIME
MANAGEMENT PITFALLS   41
Strategies to Handle Overwhelming Tasks   41
Prioritizing With ADHD: What Works and What
Doesn't   44
Managing Distractions in a Hyper-Connected World   48
The Art of Saying "No": Setting Boundaries to
Save Time   51
Avoiding and Coping With Time Management
Anxiety   53

4. LEVERAGING TECHNOLOGY FOR ENHANCED
FOCUS   57
   Apps That Work: Time Management in the
   Digital Age   58
   Gamification of Time Management Tasks   60
   Using Mind Mapping Tools for Better Task
   Organization   63
   Productivity Boosters: From Pomodoro to Time
   Blocking   66

5. EMOTIONAL INSIGHTS AND SUPPORT SYSTEMS   69
   Understanding and Managing Task-Related Anxiety   70
   The Role of Emotional Support in ADHD Time
   Management   73
   Creating a Supportive Environment at Home
   and Work   76
   Self-Motivation Techniques That Really Work
   for ADHD   78
   Dealing With Setbacks: A Resilient Approach to
   Time Management   81

6. ADVANCED STRATEGIES FOR LONG-TERM
PLANNING   87
   Mastering Long-Term Goal Setting With ADHD   88
   Breaking Down Large Projects Into Manageable
   Steps   91
   Time Management for Major Life Events   95
   Anticipating and Planning for ADHD Time
   Management Challenges   97

7. LIFESTYLE ADJUSTMENTS FOR OPTIMAL TIME
MANAGEMENT   101
   Diet, Exercise, and Sleep: The Trifecta for Better
   Focus   102
   The Impact of Physical Organization on Time
   Management   105
   Minimalism and ADHD: Reducing Clutter to
   Enhance Focus   108
   Establishing Routines That Stick: Tips and Tricks   110

8. COMMUNICATING AND COLLABORATING
WITH OTHERS   113
   Explaining Your Time Management Needs to Others   114
   Strategies for Effective Teamwork and Delegation   116

Handling Criticism and Misunderstandings About
Your Time Management   118
Building Empathy: Helping Others Understand
ADHD   121

9. TAILORING TRADITIONAL TIME MANAGEMENT
   TO FIT ADHD   125
   Customizing the Bullet Journal Approach for ADHD   126
   Time Management Myths vs. Reality for ADHD   129
   Integrating ADHD Needs Into Existing Time
   Management Systems   132
   Continuous Improvement: Evolving Your Strategies
   as Needs Change   135

10. TRANSFORMING YOUR LIFE AND
    MOTIVATIONAL INSIGHTS   139
    Time Management as a Tool for Life Transformation   139
    Establishing a Personal Time Management
    Philosophy   142
    The Future of ADHD and Time Management:
    Trends and Tools   144
    Empowering Yourself for Ongoing Success in Time
    Management   146

    Conclusion   151
    References   155

AUTHORS NOTE

Dear Reader,

Thank you for embarking on this journey to better understand time management for adults with ADHD. This book was designed with your needs in mind, focusing on delivering practical and accessible information without the distractions that can sometimes come from citations, references, or detailed instructions. As someone navigating ADHD time management hurdles, I understand how these elements can pull your attention away from the core content, making it harder to stay on task and fully absorb the material.

To help you stay focused and fully engaged with the information presented, I've intentionally kept suggestions of tools, apps, and techniques brief and straightforward. The goal is to provide you with a smooth reading experience, where the facts and strategies flow naturally, allowing you to digest the content with minimal distractions.

At the end of this book, you'll find a link to download a bonus companion work-sheets and resources workbook. This companion guide contains all the tools, apps, instructions, and additionalinformation refer-enced throughout your reading. It's there tosupport your ongoingjourney, providing the detailed instructions and references that were purposefully left out of the main text to keep you focused.

I encourage you to dive into the worksheets and resources work-book after finishing the reading. It's designed to help you take the next step—implementing what you've learned and creating your own personalized time management philosophy. With these tools in hand, you'll be better equipped to develop strategies that work for you, helping you achieve greater balance and success in time managing with ADHD.

Stay focused, stay committed, and remember that all the tools you need are just a download away at the end of your reading journey. Here's to your continued growth and success.

Warm regards,

NOELLE WALKER

READY TO DIVE IN?

I know that living with ADHD means you might feel the urge to jump ahead, to get everything you need now so you can take immediate action. And that's okay! In fact, that's part of why I've created the Companion Worksheets and Resources Workbook.

Why wait until the end of the book? You can download the workbook right now and have all the tools, apps, worksheets, and best practices ready as you read along.

Download your Bonus Companion Worksheets and Resources Workbook now. You'll get instant access to everything mentioned in the book,plus additional tools to help you on your journey to better time management with ADHD.

Take a moment now and grab it—because we all know how things can slip off the radar. Don't let this be one of them!

Simply skip to page 150 and scan the QR code or visit the link provided. We will send you a PDF copy instantly.

INTRODUCTION

Every day feels like a race against the clock, doesn't it? You wake up with a clear plan, but by noon, it feels like you're juggling flaming torches while riding a unicycle. I know this feeling all too well. Diagnosed with ADHD at the tender age of five, I've spent my life navigating the choppy waters of 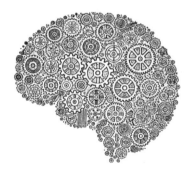 distraction, hyperactivity, and the constant battle to focus on what truly matters. If this sounds familiar, you're not alone. Many of us share these struggles; this book is a testament to our shared experiences, a reminder that we're in this together.

My journey hasn't been easy. From repeating kindergarten because I couldn't sit still to finding solace and some semblance of control in sports and kitchen timers, each chapter of my life has been a step toward understanding and managing my ADHD. I remember vividly the first time I used a kitchen timer to help me

focus on my homework. It was a game-changer. College intro-
duced new challenges, and caffeine became my best friend.
Personal, detailed study guides were my lifeline. As an adult, the
challenges persisted, and so did my determination to find effective
strategies.

This book is more than just a collection of time management
strategies. It's a testament to the struggles and successes I've experienced and an invitation for you to transform your own life. It is
written with the understanding that your mind might run a
marathon daily and offers practical, tested strategies that have
helped me lead a more focused, balanced, and fulfilling life.

This book speaks directly to you, offering empathy and practical
tools shaped to fit our unique way of experiencing the world.
From using technology to our advantage to creating environments
that enhance our ability to focus, this guide covers a range of
tactics that are not just theoretical but have been tested and proven
to work for people like us. These strategies are practical tools that
will equip you to manage your time more effectively, giving you
the confidence to take control of your day.

In these pages, you'll find a blend of personal anecdotes, practical
advice, and success stories from individuals who have walked this
path. These tales of triumph are proof of the powerful changes
that can occur when we adjust our approach to time management.
The book's structure is designed to take you from the basics of
understanding ADHD and its impact on our perception of time to
apply techniques that can significantly improve how you manage
your day.

End each day feeling like you've truly accomplished what you set
out to do. Start each morning with a clear head and a confident
heart, knowing you have the tools to tackle whatever comes your
way. Let's begin this journey together, with an open mind and a

willingness to adapt. This book is your guide, offering strategies that you can tailor to fit your unique needs and circumstances. As you take the first steps toward a more controlled, peaceful, and productive life, remember that success is within reach for adults with ADHD. With each chapter, you'll gain the tools to create a more focused, balanced, and fulfilling life. Together, we'll redefine what it means to thrive with ADHD, proving that it doesn't define us—it simply shapes how we rise to meet our challenges.

1

UNDERSTANDING ADHD AND TIME MANAGEMENT

Have you ever found yourself missing an important appointment or deadline despite having every intention to be on time? If this sounds all too familiar, you are certainly not alone. Many adults with ADHD experience similar challenges, often due to a phenomenon known as time blindness.

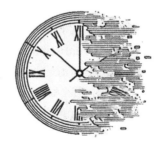

This chapter delves into the unique relationship between ADHD and time management, focusing on how intrinsic characteristics of ADHD, like time blindness, influence daily scheduling and overall productivity. By exploring these aspects, we aim to equip you with tailored strategies that align with your needs, enhancing your ability to navigate through each day more effectively.

DECODING TIME BLINDNESS IN ADHD

Time blindness is a term used to describe the difficulty in perceiving and estimating time correctly, a common issue among those with ADHD. It's about more than just being occasionally late or misjudging the duration of a task. Think of it as a pervasive difficulty that can affect every aspect of life. Simply put, it's like having a broken clock in your head. Imagine planning to take a 15-minute coffee break, only to realize an hour has passed when you thought it was just a few minutes. This isn't a simple oversight but a fundamental disconnect between the brain's internal clock and actual elapsed time.

This misalignment can significantly impact daily scheduling. Chronic lateness, missed deadlines, and underestimation of the time required for tasks are simply a few of the manifestations of time blindness. For example, you might allocate 30 minutes for a project that realistically requires 2 hours, resulting in stress, frustration, and potentially missed opportunities. The root of this issue lies in the ADHD brain's altered perception and processing of time, making time management strategies crucial for those affected.

Various practical tools and techniques can be employed to mitigate the effects of time blindness. For instance, time-tracking apps like Toggl or RescueTime help by providing external reminders of the time and duration of activities. Visual timers such as Time Timer or Timeular are another effective tool; they offer a clear and ongoing reminder of time passing, which can help pace tasks more effectively. These tools externalize time, making it more tangible and less abstract, which is particularly helpful for the ADHD mind.

Real-life applications of these strategies can be transformative. Consider the case of Alex, a graphic designer with ADHD who struggled with meeting project deadlines. By using a combination of visual timers and time-tracking software, Alex could better gauge how long tasks took and plan his workflow accordingly. This not only improved his professional performance but also reduced his daily stress levels, making work a more enjoyable and less daunting part of his life. Similarly, Sarah, a stay-at-home mom, found that using these tools helped her manage household chores more efficiently, giving her more time to spend with her children. By consistently using these tools, Alex and Sarah transformed their approach to time management, turning what was once a source of anxiety into a structured, predictable, and hopeful part of their day.

THE RELATIONSHIP BETWEEN EXECUTIVE DYSFUNCTION AND PROCRASTINATION

Executive dysfunction is a term that describes impairments in the ability to plan, organize, and execute tasks. In the context of ADHD, it's like having a faulty steering system in the complex machinery of the brain, where the gears that should be managing your tasks just don't engage properly. This often manifests as challenges with working memory, self-control, and the ability to begin and complete tasks. For anyone living with ADHD, these concepts are daily hurdles that can make even simple tasks feel overwhelming.

This dysfunction is closely tied to procrastination, a common challenge for many. Procrastination in the context of executive dysfunction isn't about laziness—it's about the real difficulty in starting tasks that demand significant mental effort. The ADHD brain can sometimes stall when asked to prioritize or sequence activities, incredibly complex or multistep tasks. Here's a simple way to visualize this: imagine your daily tasks as a series of hurdles. For someone with executive dysfunction, these aren't neatly spaced hurdles in a track meet; they're more like hurdles scattered randomly, some taller than others, some even hidden until you're right upon them. It's no wonder that getting started feels overwhelming.

We need strategies tailored to address these executive challenges to combat procrastination effectively. Breaking tasks into smaller, more manageable steps is a foundational technique. This method reduces the mental load required to start a task by making the first step small enough to be approachable. For instance, if a project seems overwhelming, beginning with a task as small as organizing your workspace or writing down the project goals can be enough to break the inertia. Another powerful strategy involves using motivational rewards. This could be as simple as treating yourself to a cup of your favorite coffee after completing some work. These rewards can create positive feedback loops that reinforce productive behavior.

Setting clear and realistic deadlines also plays a crucial role. Deadlines need to be specific but flexible enough to accommodate ADHD's unpredictable nature. Using digital calendars or task apps where reminders keep you accountable can be particularly effective. The key here is visibility and constant reminders, which help counteract ADHD's out-of-sight, out-of-mind tendency.

Let's consider a real-life example to see these strategies in action. Sandra a freelance writer with ADHD, often struggled with meeting her article submission deadlines due to procrastination stemming from executive dysfunction. By implementing a system where she broke down her writing process into clear stages— research, outline, draft, revise, and submit—she created a workflow that made the tasks seem less intimidating. Each completion of a stage earned her a small reward, ranging from a 5-minute social media break to a walk outside. Moreover, she set interim deadlines for each phase, not just the final submission. This structure not only improved her productivity but significantly reduced her work-related anxiety.

Integrating such approaches is not just about adhering to a set of rules—it's about understanding and respecting how your brain works. By doing so, you can create a personalized toolkit that mitigates the impact of executive dysfunction, turning procrastination from a regular occurrence into a manageable exception. As these methods become habits, they rebuild the faulty wiring of executive dysfunction into a more efficient system, ultimately fostering a more productive and less stressful work environment.

OVERCOMING HYPERFOCUS: BALANCING INTENSE CONCENTRATION WITH TIME AWARENESS

Hyperfocus is a common experience among individuals with ADHD, where one becomes so engrossed in a task that the world around them seems to disappear. This state of intense concentration can be a double-edged sword. On the one hand, it allows for profound engagement and extensive productivity on tasks that capture your interest. On the other, it can lead to significant disruptions in your schedule, causing you to lose track of time and neglect other essential duties or commitments. Think of hyperfocus as a superpower—an incredible ability to lock into a task with unmatched focus. Still, without proper control, letting that power steer you off course is easy.

The challenges of hyperfocus primarily revolve around its impact on time management. When you're intensely focused on a particular task, it's not just expected but typical to miss scheduled meals, ignore calls, or even skip necessary breaks, which can have repercussions on both personal and professional life. For instance, you might find yourself working on a graphic design project, so absorbed that 4 hours passed when you intended only to be working for an hour. While the progress on the project is impressive, this might mean you've missed a team meeting or haven't picked up your kids from school. This skewed perception of time can disrupt not only your plans but also affect those around you.

To manage hyperfocus effectively, consider implementing structured techniques to keep your intense concentration both beneficial and balanced. Setting alarms is a simple yet effective method to remind yourself to take breaks or move on to other tasks. For example, setting a timer for 30-minute intervals can prompt you to periodically assess whether you should continue with your current focus or redirect your attention. Scheduling hyperfocus sessions can also be incredibly beneficial—by allocating specific times in your day dedicated solely to deep focus, you can indulge in your ability to hyperfocus without letting it overrun your entire day. This method works particularly well when paired with a clear outline of what needs to be accomplished during these sessions.

Mindfulness techniques further enhance your ability to maintain an awareness of time while in a state of hyperfocus. Practicing mindfulness encourages you to stay attuned to the passage of time and your mental state, which can help you recognize when you're entering a hyperfocus mode. Simple mindfulness exercises, like pausing to take deep breaths or doing a quick body scan, can be integrated into your work sessions to keep you grounded and prevent time from slipping unnoticed.

When hyperfocus is managed correctly, it can significantly boost your productivity. Consider the story of Michael, a software developer with ADHD who struggled with missing deadlines because he became too absorbed in writing code. By implementing strategies such as setting strict time limits for his coding sessions and using apps to block out distractions, he was able to transform his hyperfocus from a liability into a powerful asset. Michael's ability to dive deep into complex problems became crucial to his success, allowing him to innovate and solve problems more effectively than many of his peers. He became known in his workplace for his creativity and ability to deliver projects on time, proving that hyperfocus can be a formidable tool in one's professional arsenal with the proper management techniques.

These approaches to balancing hyperfocus are about maintaining productivity and enhancing overall quality of life. They allow you to harness your natural tendencies and inclinations in a way that serves you rather than disrupts you. By integrating these techniques into your daily routine, you can enjoy the benefits of hyperfocus without letting it derail your day or your responsibilities. Whether through technological tools, structured scheduling, or mindful practices, taking control of your hyperfocus is about creating a framework within which your intense concentration can not only exist but thrive.

EMOTIONAL REGULATION AND ITS ROLE IN TIME MANAGEMENT

Emotional dysregulation is a familiar challenge for many with ADHD, influencing not just interpersonal relationships but also personal productivity and time management. The fluctuating emotions can often seem like a barrier that distorts our perception of time and priorities. Stress, frustration, and even excitement can skew our ability to effectively manage time, transforming what should be straightforward tasks into mountains of undue anxiety. For example, the stress from an approaching deadline might not spur action but rather a paralyzing anxiety that leads to procrastination.

Understanding the connection between emotions and time management is crucial. Emotional states heavily influence how we perceive and interact with our tasks. When emotions are not in check, everything from planning and starting a task to staying on track can become compromised. Consider the days when frustration comes from a perceived lack of progress; the natural inclination might be to abandon the task at hand, leading to further delays—essentially, a vicious cycle of emotional response and poor time management.

Addressing this requires a robust strategy for emotional regulation, which can significantly enhance time management skills. Techniques based on cognitive-behavioral therapy (CBT) are particularly effective. CBT helps in identifying and altering negative thought patterns that cause emotional distress. By learning to recognize thoughts like "I can never manage my time well" and reframing them to "Every day, I'm strengthening my time management skills," you can alleviate emotional distress and focus more on productive actions. Another practical approach is structured problem-solving, which involves breaking down perceived emotional barriers associated with specific tasks and systematically addressing them, reducing the overwhelm and making task initiation less daunting.

Relaxation exercises also play a crucial role in managing emotions. Techniques such as deep breathing, progressive muscle relaxation, or even short meditative practices can help calm the mind and reduce the impact of stress or hyperarousal on decision-making and time perception. Integrating these practices into your daily routine, particularly before commencing challenging tasks, creates a more conducive mental environment for effective time management.

The impact of improved emotional regulation on productivity is profound. By mastering control over your emotional responses, you can achieve a clearer focus, make more realistic time estimates, and approach your task list with a balanced perspective. This leads to better time management daily and contributes to long-term productivity and personal satisfaction.

Consider the transformation experienced by Lisa, a project manager who often found herself overwhelmed by the emotional stress of her job, which severely impacted her ability to meet deadlines. After incorporating relaxation exercises into her morning routine and using CBT techniques to reframe her thoughts about work-related stress, Lisa noticed a significant improvement in her productivity. She could approach her projects more calmly and with a clear mind, which improved her efficiency and allowed her to manage her time more effectively. This change did not happen overnight, but by consistently applying emotional regulation strategies, Lisa turned what was once a source of stress into a structured, manageable part of her career.

This narrative underscores the transformative power of emotional regulation in managing time more effectively. Adopting these strategies enhances your ability to deal with ADHD-related challenges and sets a foundation for sustained personal and professional growth. Whether through cognitive restructuring, relaxation techniques, or structured problem-solving, the journey toward better emotional regulation is a pivotal aspect of mastering time management with ADHD.

ADHD AND IMPULSIVITY: STRATEGIES FOR CONTROLLING SPUR-OF-THE-MOMENT DECISIONS

Impulsivity is a hallmark characteristic of ADHD, manifesting as actions taken without forethought or consideration of consequences. This trait can lead to decisions that disrupt even the best-laid plans. For example, you might impulsively decide to reorganize your office instead of working on a looming project deadline or purchase something spontaneously, throwing off your carefully planned budget. These impulsive decisions are not about lack of discipline but how the ADHD brain is wired. The neural pathways in our brains can make it challenging to resist the pull of an immediate reward or satisfaction, even when we know other, more critical tasks are at hand.

The implications of impulsivity on time management are significant. It can lead to poor allocation of time, where significant chunks of your day are spent on unplanned activities, ultimately pushing critical tasks off your schedule. This affects professional life and can strain personal relationships and self-esteem as you struggle to understand why managing time effectively is challenging. Picture this: you've planned a day to tackle a significant part of a project, but an impulsive decision to check social media spirals into hours lost. The frustration that follows can be overwhelming, not just for you but for those depending on your contributions.

Controlling this impulsivity involves a combination of awareness, structure, and tools. Planning tools such as digital calendars, specialized ADHD apps, or traditional planners can help establish a more structured day. You can create a routine that makes impulsive decisions less likely by clearly outlining what needs to be done and allocating specific times for these tasks. These tools work best when regularly updated and reviewed, making them a central part of your daily management strategy.

Impulse control training is another effective strategy. Techniques like delayed gratification, where you train yourself to wait for a bigger reward instead of succumbing to the immediate urge, can be very beneficial. This could be as simple as setting a rule where you only check your phone after completing a task, not during. Additionally, setting up accountability systems—whether through apps that track your behavior and provide feedback or through a trusted friend or coach who checks in on your progress—can provide the external motivation needed to manage impulsive tendencies.

Success stories abound where individuals have turned their impulsive traits into managed behaviors, contributing to effective time management. Take the case of James, a freelance graphic designer known for his creative genius but plagued by his inability to meet deadlines due to impulsive habits. By using a digital planner that mapped out every hour of his workday and setting short-term goals that he could tick off for satisfaction, James was able to curb his impulsiveness. He aligned his need for immediate gratification with productive activities that also contributed to his ultimate goals. Over time, this helped him meet deadlines and build a reputation for reliability, starkly contrasting his previous track record.

Another example is Maria, a college student who struggled with impulsive spending and time management. She started using an app that tracked her spending and how she spent her time, linking the two to show how unplanned activities affected her budget and study hours. This visual representation helped Maria see the direct consequences of her impulsiveness. With the help of a mentor, she set up weekly reviews to evaluate her progress, adjusting her strategies as needed. This ongoing process not only improved her financial stability but also her academic performance.

When it comes to managing impulsivity, the goal isn't to suppress your spontaneous traits completely but to channel them into productive avenues that don't derail your time management efforts. The strategies discussed here provide a framework for understanding and molding your impulsive tendencies into a structured form that enhances productivity rather than hinders it. By consistently applying these methods, you can transform impulsivity from a disruptive force into a controlled energy that propels you toward your goals.

As we navigate the complexities of ADHD and time management, remember that each step taken toward controlling impulsivity is a step toward greater personal and professional fulfillment. The techniques and tools merely aid you in harnessing the full potential of your vibrant, dynamic personality. Through persistent effort and dedication, managing time effectively while accommodating your natural inclinations isn't just possible; with time, it becomes a sustainable part of your life.

2

CUSTOM TOOLS AND TECHNIQUES FOR EVERYDAY PRODUCTIVITY

Imagine stepping into a workshop with tools uniquely tailored for you, each designed to your specific needs and preferences. This chapter is just like that, offering bespoke tools to enhance daily productivity. Here, we explore the vital role of a well-structured daily planner, a cornerstone tool for anyone, espe- 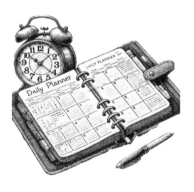 cially if navigating the dynamic waters of ADHD. A planner isn't just about keeping dates—it's about creating a roadmap that aligns with how your mind works, helping you harness your strengths and mitigate your challenges.

DESIGNING YOUR ADHD-FRIENDLY DAILY PLANNER

Creating a planner that caters to the ADHD mind requires understanding that traditional planning methods might not always align with your needs. For those with ADHD, a planner isn't just a place to jot down dates and tasks—it becomes a flexible tool that adjusts to your changing focus and motivation. The importance of this customization cannot be overstated—it transforms a standard organizational tool into something that feels like a part of your cognitive process, making managing tasks less of a battle and more of a seamless integration into your daily life.

Key Features to Include

First, let's discuss the essential features that make a planner ADHD-friendly. Color coding is a fantastic way to manage visual attention. For example, you might use blue for work-related tasks, green for personal errands, and yellow for appointments. This method makes your planner easier to scan and leverages color psychology to help you mentally organize and prioritize tasks more effectively. Another crucial feature is clear sections for prioritization. This could have a dedicated space at the top or side of each page where you can list high-priority tasks that need immediate attention. Finally, flexibility is critical. Your planner should allow you to adjust tasks easily—whether that means shifting them to another day or breaking them into smaller, more manageable parts. This adaptability is crucial for dealing with the often unpredictable nature of ADHD, where you might find your ability to tackle specific tasks changes from day to day.

Integration With Digital Tools

Integrating digital tools with traditional planners in today's tech-driven world can significantly enhance functionality and accessibility. Many digital planning tools offer beneficial features for ADHD, such as customizable reminders, recurring tasks, and the ability to sync across multiple devices. This integration allows you to maintain the tactile benefits of writing in a planner while enjoying the dynamic capabilities of digital tools. For instance, you could use a digital app to send reminders to your phone about upcoming tasks, which are also written in your physical planner. This dual approach ensures that you have multiple cues to help keep you on track, catering to the ADHD brain's need for external stimuli to maintain focus.

Examples of Effective Planners

To illustrate, let's consider the example of Emily, a digital marketer with ADHD who struggled to track her multiple projects and deadlines. Emily switched to a planner that allowed for color coding and included a digital component, which she could access from her smartphone and computer. She used different colors for each project and set digital reminders for each phase of her marketing campaigns. This system helped her stay organized and significantly reduced her anxiety, as she could visually see her week at a glance and adjust her schedule as needed without feeling overwhelmed.

Another example is Mark, a freelance graphic designer, who found that traditional planners never suited his workflow. He opted for a custom-designed digital planner that allowed him to set irregular reminder intervals—aligned with his variable work hours—and included a digital sketchpad to jot down ideas as they came to him. This blend of planning and creative space was crucial for him, as it catered to the spontaneous nature of his creativity while keeping him anchored to his daily tasks and responsibilities.

These examples vividly illustrate the transformative impact of a well-designed ADHD-friendly planner on managing daily tasks and enhancing overall productivity. Whether it's through color-coding, prioritization, or a combination of digital tools, a customized planner can effectively address the unique challenges posed by ADHD. It can turn daily planning from a dreaded chore into an empowering routine that complements your workflow and cognitive style. Using a planner tailored to your needs can give you a sense of control and capability, knowing you have the tools to manage your day effectively.

TIME BLINDNESS TECHNIQUES FOR THE ADHD MIND

Navigating the day can sometimes feel like trying to solve a puzzle where the pieces don't quite fit. For those of us with ADHD, the concept of time often eludes our grasp, not because we aren't aware of its importance but because our perception of it can be fundamentally different. This discrepancy in how we experience time can lead to various challenges, from underestimating how long a task will take to feeling like time is slipping through our fingers without tangible achievement. To bridge this gap, specialized techniques for estimating time can become invaluable tools in our daily lives.

Understanding the nuances of time perception among individuals with ADHD is crucial. Often, we might experience what is known as "time inconsistency," where our internal clock doesn't quite align with the actual passage of time. This can mean thinking that 5 minutes have passed when, in reality, it has been 20. It's more than just a minor miscalculation—it impacts how we plan our days, meet deadlines, and manage responsibilities. The need for specialized blindness techniques arises from this challenge, aiming to provide a scaffold that aligns our perception more closely with real-time. Knowing that you're not alone in this struggle, and that others share the same challenges, can provide a sense of validation, connection, and make you feel more understood and less isolated in your journey with ADHD. Acknowledging the anxiety that can come from feeling like time is slipping away is also important.

We'll discuss strategies for managing this anxiety later in the chapter.

Adopting practical strategies for time blindness can significantly enhance how effectively you manage your day. One technique involves using historical task timing data. You can better understand your time needs by keeping a log of how long it takes to complete various tasks. This log can be as simple as a notebook entry or as detailed as a spreadsheet. For instance, if you record that writing a report takes 4 hours rather than the 2 you initially thought, you can plan better for future reports.

Another strategy is breaking larger tasks into smaller, more manageable components. This makes the task seem less daunting and allows for more precise time allocation to each segment. If you estimate a project will take 10 hours, break it down into smaller tasks like research, writing, editing, and final review, assigning a time estimate to each. This breakdown provides a more precise roadmap to completion and prevents individuals from being overwhelmed, often leading to procrastination. Knowing that you have the tools to break down tasks and manage your time effectively is empowering, giving you a sense of control and reducing feeling overwhelmed.

Incorporating software tools designed for time blindness can also play a pivotal role. Many digital tools offer features like time tracking, reminders, and even predictive time blindness based on past task durations. These tools take much of the guesswork out of planning your day, providing a structured framework that can help counteract the natural time inconsistency experienced by many with ADHD.

To bring these concepts to life, consider the story of Jenna, a web developer who often worked late into the night, struggling to meet deadlines. She began to use a time-tracking app to record how long each coding session lasted and what parts of her projects were consuming the most time. This data helped her identify areas where she needed to improve efficiency and also helped in setting more realistic deadlines with her clients. Over time, Jenna's ability to estimate project times improved, and she found herself feeling less stressed and more in control of her workload.

Training Exercises: Time Trials and Reflective Journaling

Engaging in specific exercises can be highly beneficial for further refining your time-blindness skills. Time trials, for example, involve estimating how long you think a task will take before you begin and timing yourself as you do it. This exercise helps calibrate your internal clock to be more in sync with actual time. Start with daily tasks, like reading emails or preparing meals, and gradually work up to more complex projects.

Reflective journaling is another powerful tool. At the end of each day, take a few minutes to compare your time estimates to the actual time spent on tasks. This reflection can provide insights into patterns of under or overestimation and help you adjust your approach accordingly. For instance, you may notice that creative tasks take longer than anticipated, suggesting a need to allocate more time for these in the future.

By incorporating these techniques and exercises into your routine, you can develop a more accurate sense of time, which is essential for effective time management in both personal and professional contexts. As you become more adept at estimating how long tasks will take, you'll find it easier to plan your days, meet deadlines, and reduce stress, leading to a more productive and balanced life.

SETTING UP EFFECTIVE REMINDERS AND ALARMS

In the fast-paced rhythm of daily life, especially when navigating the complexities of ADHD, setting up effective reminders and alarms can be akin to having a personal assistant by your side, gently nudging you toward your next task or commitment. The right tools and strategies for setting reminders can significantly alter how you manage your time and tasks, turning potential oversights into completed actions. Let's explore the tools available, how to customize them to fit your unique needs, and understand their profound impact on your daily productivity and mental well-being.

Selecting the appropriate tools for reminders is crucial. In our digital age, the options are vast, ranging from smartphone apps that offer various notification options to traditional timers that provide a physical presence reminding you of passing time. Smartphone apps are versatile, offering features tailored to different needs and preferences. For instance, you can choose apps that allow you to set multiple alarms throughout the day, which can be particularly useful for segmenting work tasks or reminding you to take necessary breaks. On the other hand, traditional timers, such as kitchen timers or even hourglasses, provide a tangible reminder of time's passage, which can be genuinely grounding for some.

Customization of these tools is critical to making them work effectively for you. One powerful customization option is varying alarm tones. By assigning different tones to different types of tasks or reminders—such as a gentle tone for a reminder to take a break and a more urgent tone for a work deadline—you can subconsciously associate specific sounds with specific actions, enhancing your response to these cues. The strategic placement of alarms is another critical consideration. For instance, placing a physical timer where you frequently pass by, such as next to your coffee machine or on your desk, ensures that you are regularly reminded of the passing time without needing to check a device. Timing your reminders is also crucial; setting them to go off a few minutes before you need to start a new task can give you enough time to mentally prepare and shift gears, which is especially helpful if you tend to hyperfocus.

The psychological impact of well-timed and well-placed reminders is profound. For individuals with ADHD, the day can sometimes feel like a blur of activities that are difficult to keep track of, which can lead to anxiety and a sense of being over-whelmed. Effective reminders can mitigate these feelings by providing external cues that help structure your day and reduce the cognitive load of remembering every scheduled detail. This can lower anxiety levels and increase your ability to focus on the task at hand, knowing that you will be appropriately prompted when it's time to move on to the next activity. Moreover, these reminders help reinforce a sense of control and competence, which can be significantly empowering.

To illustrate the transformative impact of effective reminder systems, consider the story of Clara, a freelance writer with ADHD who often struggled with time management, particularly in balancing writing with her other responsibilities like appoint-ments and family commitments. Clara started using a smartphone app that allowed her to set custom alarms for different tasks, each with unique tones that she chose based on the nature of the task. She also used a traditional clock with a loud alarm in her work-space to remind her when to finish her current task and begin another. This combination of digital and physical reminders helped her stay on schedule without feeling overwhelmed. Over time, Clara reported a significant reduction in her daily stress levels and improved ability to meet deadlines and manage her day.

She found that the reminders acted as cues for action and reassurances that she wouldn't let anything slip through the cracks, allowing her to focus more fully on the task without the nagging worry of forgetting something important.

Incorporating effective reminder systems into your daily routine can thus be a game-changer, particularly when navigating the challenges of ADHD. By choosing the right tools, customizing them to suit your needs, and understanding their psychological benefits, you can create a structured yet flexible framework that supports your productivity and reduces anxiety. Whether through digital apps, traditional timers, or a combination of both, setting up effective reminders is about crafting a personal strategy that respects your cognitive style and enhances your ability to manage time and tasks efficiently.

THE ROLE OF VISUAL AIDS IN MANAGING TIME

Visual aids can be a game-changer in overcoming time blindness and enhancing task management, particularly for individuals with ADHD. These are tangible markers of time and tasks, grounding abstract concepts into visible, manageable forms. They transform the concept of time from an elusive idea into something you can see and interact with, which can dramatically improve your ability to manage it effectively.

Let's explore how these tools can be integrated into your daily life to provide structure and clarity. One of the simplest yet most effective visual aids is the wall calendar. It provides a constant visual reminder of scheduled tasks and appointments, which can be crucial for someone with ADHD. Placing a large wall calendar in a frequently used area, such as your kitchen or office, lets you keep track of daily activities at a glance. Another powerful visual aid is the Gantt chart, which is handy for more complex projects involving multiple tasks and deadlines. Gantt charts help visualize the project timeline and understand how various tasks overlap and relate to each other, making it easier to manage large projects without feeling overwhelmed.

GANTT CHART

Task name	Q1 2022			Q2 2022		Q3 2022	Assignees
	Jan-22	Feb-22	Mar-22	Apr-22	Jun-22	Jul-22	
Enhancements							SKD
Designing							KNR
Implementation							NK, SG
Testing							SG DK
Fixing bugs and final release							SKD, KNR

Digital dashboards represent another category of visual aids, harnessing technology to track multiple tasks and deadlines effectively. These dashboards can be customized to display important information such as upcoming deadlines, daily tasks, and time spent on each activity. This real-time feedback is invaluable for staying on track and adjusting as needed.

Implementing these visual aids into your daily planning involves a few key steps. First, identify where you need the most help—keeping track of daily tasks, managing a project, or simply remembering appointments. Choose the visual aid that best suits your needs; for instance, a wall calendar for daily activities or a Gantt chart for project work.

Once you've selected the appropriate tool, position it where you often see it. This could be on your desk, by the front door, or as the homepage on your digital devices. Regular interaction with your visual aid is crucial; make it a habit to check and update it at least once a day. This could be in the morning as you plan your day or in the evening as you prepare for the next day. Over time, these visual aids will become an integral part of your routine, providing a reliable structure to help manage your time and tasks more effectively.

The impact of visual aids on time management for individuals with ADHD can be profound, as demonstrated in several case studies. Consider the example of Tom, a software developer who struggled with meeting project deadlines. His work often involves complex tasks that can be overwhelming, leading to procrastination and last-minute rushes. Using a Gantt chart, Tom could break his projects into smaller, more manageable tasks and set realistic deadlines. The visual representation of his project timelines helped him stay on track and significantly reduced his workplace stress.

Another case is Anna, a college student with ADHD who found it challenging to balance her coursework, part-time job, and social life. She started using apps as a digital dashboard helping her visualize how she spent her time daily. This enabled her to allocate time more effectively and made her more mindful of how she used her time. As a result, Anna strengthened her time management skills, leading to better school performance and less anxiety about her schedule.

These examples highlight the transformative potential of visual aids in managing time, particularly for individuals with ADHD. By making the abstract concept of time more concrete and visually accessible, these tools can help you better understand and control how you spend your days. Whether through simple wall calendars, detailed Gantt charts, or interactive digital dashboards, integrating visual aids into your time management strategy can significantly improve productivity and reduce stress, making your daily life more structured and predictable.

BUILDING ROUTINE WITH ADHD: A STEP-BY-STEP GUIDE

Establishing a routine when you have ADHD can sometimes feel like trying to pin the tail on a moving donkey—challenging, often frustrating, but not impossible. The importance of a consistent routine cannot be overstated, especially for those of us with ADHD. It serves as a framework that reduces the number of decisions we need to make about our daily activities, thereby decreasing the cognitive load and minimizing the chances of becoming overwhelmed or distracted. Essentially, a solid routine can free up mental space and energy for focusing on the tasks at hand, leading to improved time management and productivity.

To build a routine that sticks, start by understanding your personal rhythms and preferences. Are you a morning person, or do you find your stride in the evening? Aligning your routine with your natural inclinations rather than working against them can make sticking to it much easier and more productive. Begin by identifying the tasks that you need to accomplish daily, such as taking medication, working, studying, or exercising. Then, schedule consistent times for these activities based on when you are usually most alert and focused. For instance, if you are most energized in the morning, schedule your most challenging tasks during this time.

Next, create a visual representation of your routine. This could be a detailed timetable on a whiteboard, a digital calendar, or even a simple list on your fridge. Seeing your routine laid out visually helps solidify it in your mind and allows you to assess when you have spare time or are overbooked quickly. It's crucial, however, to build in flexibility. The unpredictable nature of ADHD means that some days will be easier than others. The ability to shift tasks around as needed without disrupting your entire routine is essential for maintaining long-term adherence.

One common barrier to sticking to a routine is the need for immediate motivation. To overcome this, tie specific, immediate rewards to completing tasks within your routine. For example, allow yourself a few minutes of social media after finishing a work session or treat yourself to a favorite snack after a workout. These small incentives can make completing routine tasks more appealing and satisfying, boosting your motivation to stick with your schedule.

Another challenge is managing external distractions, derailing even the most well-planned routine. Minimize distractions by setting boundaries with others and creating an environment conducive to focus. This can be achieved either by using noise-canceling headphones while working, turning off non-essential notifications on your devices, or having a clear signal, like a closed door, that tells others you need uninterrupted time. Regularly reviewing and adjusting your routine is also essential. As your responsibilities, interests, and skills change, so should your routine. Monthly or quarterly reviews help ensure your routine meets your goals and needs.

Let's consider the example of Julia, a graphic artist with ADHD who struggled to meet client deadlines due to her sporadic work habits. By establishing a routine that designated specific times for brainstorming, designing, client communication, and administrative tasks, Julia could create a balanced workflow that accommodated her creative needs while ensuring she stayed on top of her responsibilities. She used a digital calendar with alerts to remind her of task transitions and built-in short breaks to prevent burnout. This new structured approach improved her productivity and her client relationship, leading to more repeat business and less stress.

Another success story is Ben, a high school teacher with ADHD, who found that a lack of routine led to ungraded papers piling up and lesson plans being prepared at the last minute. He decided to set specific times for grading and planning immediately after school hours, using the momentum of the workday to keep him going. He also instituted a "power hour" where he focused entirely on tasks he disliked, using a timer to count down. This helped him keep his job responsibilities in check and improved his evenings and weekends, making them more relaxing and enjoyable.

These examples highlight how personalized, well-structured routines can significantly enhance day-to-day functioning and overall life satisfaction for individuals with ADHD. By developing a routine that works for you and being prepared to adapt it as necessary, you can create a powerful tool that supports your productivity and personal goals.

In wrapping up this chapter, it's clear that building and maintaining a routine when you have ADHD involves a blend of self-awareness, strategic planning, and flexibility. The process requires you to understand your needs, set up structures that guide you, and adjust as necessary, but the rewards—increased productivity, reduced stress, and a greater sense of control over your life—are well worth the effort. As we move forward, remember that each step you take in refining your routine is a step toward a more organized and fulfilling life.

3

TACKLING COMMON ADHD TIME MANAGEMENT PITFALLS

Imagine you're about to climb a mountain. From the base, it looks impossible, towering, and over-whelming. But then, you learn about a path carved out by those who ventured before you. This path breaks the journey into manageable segments, each leading safely to the next until, before you know it, 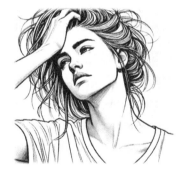 you're at the peak. Managing large tasks with ADHD can feel just as daunting as climbing a mountain, but just like that, the right strategies can make the journey achievable and enjoyable.

STRATEGIES TO HANDLE OVERWHELMING TASKS

When faced with a big project or task, the initial wave of motivation often gives way to a sense of overwhelm, especially when your ADHD brain struggles to find a starting point. Breaking tasks into manageable pieces is not just about making things more accessible;

it's about changing how you interact with your tasks, transforming them from sources of stress into sources of success.

Breaking Tasks Into Manageable Pieces

Breaking tasks into smaller components is a relief for the ADHD brain. Large, undefined tasks can lead to cognitive overload, a common issue for those with ADHD. This relief is not just a theoretical concept; it's a practical benefit that can significantly improve your ability to manage tasks. By dividing an enormous task into smaller, more manageable steps, you create achievable goals and reduce the mental strain that often accompanies the planning and execution of complex tasks.

For example, if you're tasked with organizing a major event, break it down into categories like venue booking, guest invitations, and catering. Each category can then be broken down further. For venue booking, the steps include researching venues, visiting potential sites, and then making a reservation. Similarly, you can break down guest invitations into creating a guest list, designing and sending invitations, and managing RSVPs. This systematic breakdown makes the process more digestible and provides clear action points that help maintain focus and momentum.

Use of Visual Task Maps

Visual task maps are a powerful tool in your strategy arsenal. They allow you to lay out the broken-down tasks visually, making it easier to see how they connect and what needs to be prioritized. More than just a planning tool, these maps offer a sense of control and empowerment over your tasks, guiding you through your work and significantly reducing the feeling of being overwhelmed.

Creating a visual task map can be as simple as drawing circles (nodes) for each task on paper and connecting them with lines to show the relationship and flow between tasks. Digital tools like Lucidchart or MindMeister offer more sophisticated options like adding deadlines and collaborators or attaching files directly to each node.

Establishing Clear Milestones

Setting clear, achievable milestones within larger tasks is crucial. Milestones act as checkpoints that help to gauge progress and provide opportunities for evaluation and adjustment without waiting until the task's end. They are instrumental in maintaining motivation, as each milestone is a small victory, reinforcing your progress.

For instance, in the event organization example, a milestone could be the confirmation of the venue booking. Reaching this milestone marks progress and solidifies the foundation for subsequent tasks. Celebrating these small wins is a crucial part of the process. They prove that you are moving forward and help keep morale high. This celebration can bring a sense of motivation and encouragement, making the task seem more manageable.

Leveraging Technology

Technology can significantly streamline the process of managing complex tasks. Several apps are designed specifically to cater to the needs of individuals with ADHD. These tools can help break down tasks, set reminders for deadlines, and even block out distractions.

Project management software—like Trello, Asana, or Monday.com —allows you to create task boards where each project component can be monitored, updated, and shared with team members. These tools often include features like setting due dates, adding comments, and integrating other services like email or cloud storage, which can be extremely helpful in keeping all your information and communication in one place.

Consider the case of Oliver, a digital marketer managing multiple client projects simultaneously. Using a project management tool, he created separate boards for each client, with tasks categorized by urgency and complexity. This helped him stay organized and made communicating progress to his clients easier, enhancing transparency and trust.

Incorporating these strategies into your workflow can transform overwhelming tasks into small, manageable actions. Like climbing a mountain, the key is to take one step at a time, using the best tools and strategies to reach the summit successfully. As you apply these methods, remember that each small step is a progress point, bringing you closer to your goal, reducing stress, and increasing your efficiency and productivity.

PRIORITIZING WITH ADHD: WHAT WORKS AND WHAT DOESN'T

Prioritizing tasks effectively is crucial, especially when your brain's executive functions are already stretched. For adults with ADHD, the challenge isn't choosing what to do first but consistently making decisions that align with long-term goals rather than immediate gratification or current mood.

THE EISENHOWER BOX

	URGENT	NOT URGENT
IMPORTANT	**DO** Do it now. Write article for today.	**DECIDE** Schedule a time to do it. Exercising. Calling family and friends. Researching articles. Long-term biz strategy.
NOT IMPORTANT	**DELEGATE** Who can do it for you? Scheduling interviews. Booking flights. Approving comments. Answering certain emails. Sharing articles.	**DELETE** Eliminate it. Watching television. Checking social media. Sorting through junk mail.

"What is important is seldom urgent and what is urgent is seldom important."
-Dwight Eisenhower, 34th President of the United States

Effective prioritization requires a straightforward method for assessing the importance and urgency of each task. This assessment is often visualized through tools like the Eisenhower Box, which divides tasks into four categories based on their urgency and importance. The four categories are (a) urgent and important, (b) important but not urgent, (c) urgent but not important, and (d) neither urgent nor important. Tasks that are urgent and important should be tackled first, while those that are neither urgent nor important might not need your attention.

Creating a daily list of tasks and applying this categorization can help clarify which actions require immediate attention and which can be planned for later. However, it's crucial to remain flexible as the day's events might shift what becomes urgent. For someone with ADHD, this flexibility, paired with a clear structure, can prevent the feeling of being overwhelmed. Limiting the number of top-priority tasks is also beneficial to avoid cognitive fatigue. Focusing on three primary daily tasks can keep you productive without feeling overloaded.

The pitfalls in prioritization often stem from common ADHD traits such as impulsivity or hyperfocus on less critical tasks that might be more enjoyable or provide immediate satisfaction. Overcommitting is another frequent challenge, where the optimistic estimation of one's available energy and time leads to an unmanageable packed schedule. Recognizing these tendencies is the first step in mitigating their effects. Reviewing your commitments regularly and assessing whether each aligns with your larger goals is advantageous. If a task or project doesn't serve a clear purpose, it might be time to reconsider its priority or delegate it.

Daily Prioritization Exercises

Incorporating specific exercises into your routine can be immensely helpful for honing prioritization skills. One practical approach is evening reflection combined with morning planning. Each evening, take a few minutes to reflect on the day: what tasks were completed, which were delayed, and any new tasks that have emerged. This reflection helps you understand your productivity patterns and any recurrent distractions or unnecessary commitments.

In the morning, use your insights from the evening before to plan your day. Write down your top three priorities based on urgency and importance. This sets a clear focus and helps mentally prepare for the tasks ahead. Over time, this practice can improve your ability to estimate how much you can realistically achieve in a day, reducing feelings of frustration and inefficiency.

Using Tools for Prioritization

Leveraging technology can significantly enhance your ability to prioritize effectively. Numerous apps and tools are designed to assist with task management and prioritization. Priority matrix apps, for example, allow you to categorize tasks according to different criteria, making it easier to see at a glance what you should focus on next. These apps often include features like due dates, reminders, and progress tracking, which can help keep you on track.

Another helpful tool is priority cards. These are simple, physical cards where you can write down your tasks and rearrange them as needed throughout the day. Having a tangible representation of your tasks that you can manipulate can be especially helpful for visual thinkers. It also provides a satisfying physical action to accompany completing a task, such as moving a card from the "to do" section to the "done" section, which can be rewarding and motivating.

Incorporating these strategies into your daily life improves your productivity and enhances your sense of control and satisfaction with your work. Prioritization is not just about getting things done; it's about ensuring you're getting the right things done in order, which can make all the difference in managing ADHD effectively. By assessing the importance and urgency of your tasks, avoiding common pitfalls, practicing daily prioritization, and utilizing helpful tools, you can create a tailored approach that enhances your focus and productivity, allowing you to achieve more with less stress.

MANAGING DISTRACTIONS IN A HYPER-CONNECTED WORLD

In the digital age, where information and communication bombard us incessantly, managing distractions has become a crucial skill, particularly for adults with ADHD. Distractions can significantly impede your ability to focus and get things done, turning what should be a productive day into a series of uncompleted tasks and frustrations. Understanding and mitigating these distractions starts with a deep dive into what explicitly pulls your attention away.

Identifying Personal Distraction Triggers

The first step in mastering your environment and mind's wandering tendencies is identifying your personal distraction triggers. Distractions can be external, like phone notifications and background noise, or internal, such as daydreaming or emotional disturbances.

Start by keeping a distraction log. Each time you find yourself drifting away from a task, jot down what caused it, the time, and what you were working on. Over a week, patterns will likely emerge. You might notice, for example, that social media notifications lure you away from your work more often than you realize or that you tend to lose focus mid-afternoon when your energy dips.

This log provides an eye-opener to the specific conditions and stimuli that disrupt your focus. With this knowledge, you can create targeted strategies to mitigate these distractions. For instance, if you're most distracted by emails, you might close your email client for uninterrupted work periods, checking it only at designated times.

Strategies to Minimize Digital Distractions

Digital distractions are among the most pervasive and disruptive, with their constant pings pulling your attention away from tasks that require depth and concentration. One effective strategy to combat this is using website and app blockers. Tools like Freedom or Cold Turkey allow you to block distracting websites and apps during work hours, freeing you from the temptation to scroll through social media or check the news.

Setting boundaries on smartphone use is also crucial. This can include keeping your phone in another room while you work or using features like "Do Not Disturb" during critical work periods. Customizing notifications so that only the most important ones come through can also reduce the constant interruption. For example, you might set your phone to only alert you for direct messages or calls from critical contacts, ensuring you're not disturbed by every app or social media notification.

Creating a Distraction-Free Environment

Your physical environment plays a significant role in how well you can focus. Creating a workspace that minimizes distractions can significantly enhance your productivity. Start with your desk. Keep it organized and precise of unnecessary items. Each extra item on your desk can act as a potential distraction. Next, consider your lighting and noise levels. Natural light is ideal, but if possible, ensure your lighting is not too harsh or dim, as poor lighting can strain your eyes and distract you. Noise can be trickier, especially in busy environments. Noise-canceling headphones can be a lifesaver in these situations, or you might find that background music or white noise helps mask disruptive sounds.

Mindfulness and Focus Training Techniques

Training your mind to resist distractions is another powerful strategy. Mindfulness exercises can enhance your ability to concentrate and remain present in the moment. Simple practices like focused breathing or meditation can be done in just a few minutes but have long-lasting effects on your ability to focus. Apps like Headspace or Calm offer guided meditations specifically designed to improve concentration.

Focus training exercises can also be beneficial. For example, the Pomodoro Technique, developed in the late 1980s, involves breaking your workday into 25-minute chunks of focused work time, followed by five5-minute breaks. These intervals are known as 'Pomodoros'"Pomodoros." After completing four Pomodoros, you take a longer break of about 15 to 30 minutes. This method is particularly beneficial because it aligns well with the concentration spans of many adults with ADHD, who might find prolonged focus challenging. It helps by creating a rhythm that promotes sustained concentration and ensures regular breaks to prevent burnout.

By implementing these strategies, you can create an environment and a mindset that helps shield you from the myriad distractions of our modern world. Keeping a log helps maintain awareness of what disrupts your focus, while tools and techniques for minimizing distractions support maintaining that focus. Together, they empower you to control your attention rather than being at the mercy of every notification and environmental disturbance.

THE ART OF SAYING "NO": SETTING BOUNDARIES TO SAVE TIME

Recognizing the need to set boundaries and comfortably say no can be transformative, especially for those with ADHD who might find themselves routinely overwhelmed by over-commitment. Establishing boundaries is about knowing your limits and communicating them clearly to others. This practice protects your time and energy and significantly reduces stress by preventing you from taking on more than you can handle. It's about making conscious choices on what to accept and what to decline so that you can prioritize effectively without feeling stretched too thin.

For many with ADHD, the challenge often lies in the fear of missing out or disappointing others, which can lead to saying yes to almost everything. However, this over-commitment can lead to a cycle of stress and burnout, which hampers productivity and affects overall well-being. Therefore, assessing each request or commitment that comes your way is crucial by asking whether it aligns with your priorities and whether you realistically have the time and energy to commit to it. This assessment should be guided by clearly understanding your personal and professional goals and a realistic evaluation of your current workload and individual energy levels.

Practical Ways to Say "No"

Telling the person in a polite way there is no need to be confrontational or negative can be done gracefully and assertively, ensuring your relationships remain intact. Here are some phrases that can help you say "no" effectively:

- "I appreciate you thinking of me for this, but I can't commit to it at the moment."
- "I'm currently focusing on some priorities that need my full attention, so I won't be able to take this on."
- "I need to pass on this right now, but please keep me in mind for future opportunities."
- "I don't have the bandwidth to give this the attention it deserves right now."

Using these phrases can help you communicate your decision clearly and respectfully, showing that your refusal is not a matter of unwillingness but instead of prioritizing your commitments to ensure you can deliver quality results where you have chosen to focus.

Role-Playing Scenarios

Practicing how to say "no" can make it easier when real situations arise. Role-playing scenarios with a friend or mentor can be particularly effective. For instance, imagine a scenario where a colleague asks you to take on an extra project when you already have a full schedule. Practice how you would convey your inability to take on more work using the phrases above. Your practice partner can offer feedback on your delivery, helping you find the right balance between politeness and assertiveness.

Balancing Flexibility and Firmness

While being firm in your boundaries is essential, maintaining flexibility is equally important. Life is unpredictable, and being too rigid in your boundaries can lead to missed opportunities or strained relationships. The key is to evaluate each situation independently and determine where a little flexibility could lead to a beneficial outcome without causing undue stress or distraction.

For instance, if a high-priority opportunity conflicts with less critical tasks, it might be worth rearranging your commitments. However, this flexibility should not lead you to compromise on your non-negotiables, such as family time or personal downtime. It's about making informed adjustments aligning with your priorities and values.

By mastering the art of saying "no" and setting effective boundaries, you can take a significant step toward better managing your time and energy. This practice helps reduce the feeling of being overwhelmed and enhances your ability to focus on your goals with greater clarity and commitment. Remember, every "no" you say to something that doesn't fit your priorities is a "yes" to something that does. This mindset shift is crucial in helping you stay true to your path and ensure that your actions align with your personal and professional aspirations.

AVOIDING AND COPING WITH TIME MANAGEMENT ANXIETY

Time management anxiety is a natural and often overwhelming experience for many adults with ADHD. It's that gnawing feeling in your stomach when you think about the day ahead or the palpable tension that builds up as you face your to-do list.

Recognizing the symptoms of this anxiety is the first step toward managing it effectively. Common signs include restlessness, irritability, and procrastination, particularly when planning or starting tasks. You might also experience physical symptoms such as headaches or an increased heart rate when thinking about managing your time or upcoming deadlines.

Understanding what triggers your anxiety is crucial. It could be triggered by a looming deadline, a packed schedule, or even the thought of organizing your day. Once you are aware of these triggers, you can begin to apply specific techniques to manage your reactions and reduce anxiety levels.

Techniques to Reduce Anxiety

Several techniques can be instrumental in managing time management anxiety. Deep breathing exercises are a simple yet effective method to calm your mind and body. When you start feeling overwhelmed, focus on your breathing for a few moments. Breathe slowly through your nose, hold for a few seconds, and exhale slowly through your mouth. This helps reduce the "fight-or-flight" response that anxiety triggers and can bring a sense of calm to your mind, making it easier to focus.

Progressive muscle relaxation is another technique that can help. This involves tensing each muscle group in your body for a few seconds and then relaxing them. This process not only helps in relieving the physical symptoms of stress and anxiety but also shifts your focus away from anxiety-inducing thoughts.

Positive self-talk can also make a significant difference. This involves consciously shifting negative or anxious thoughts to more positive, constructive ones. For instance, replacing thoughts like "I can never get this done on time" with "I have managed similar tasks before, and I can manage this too" can help alleviate anxiety and boost your confidence.

Planning and Preparation Strategies

Thorough planning and preparation play a pivotal role in mitigating anxiety related to time management. The uncertainty of what lies ahead can often be a significant anxiety trigger. By creating a detailed plan or schedule, you can give yourself a clear roadmap of what needs to be done, which can significantly reduce feelings of anxiety.

Daily, weekly, or monthly planning templates help streamline the process and ensure consistency. These templates should include time blocks for specific tasks—built-in buffers for unexpected events—and breaks to prevent burnout. Visual planning tools, such as calendars or planners with color coding, can also help make your schedule easy to understand at a glance, which helps reduce the anxiety that comes from feeling disorganized.

Seeking Professional Help

While these techniques and strategies can be highly effective, there are times when time management anxiety might feel too over-whelming to handle on your own. In such cases, seeking support from a mental health professional is a wise step.

Anxiety is a common issue that can be managed with the right help, and there is no shame in seeking assistance. Therapists can provide you with personalized strategies and tools to manage your anxiety more effectively. They can also help you explore under-lying issues that might be contributing to your anxiety, offering a comprehensive approach to managing your symptoms.

Remember, coping with time management anxiety is not about eliminating anxiety completely but about learning how to control and direct it so that it does not hinder your productivity or well-being. By recognizing the symptoms, employing effective tech-niques, planning thoroughly, and seeking help when needed, you can transform your anxiety from a barrier into a manageable aspect of your life, allowing you to focus more on achieving your goals and less on the stress that comes with trying to manage your time.

As we conclude this chapter, remember that managing time effectively with ADHD involves practical strategies for organizing tasks and emotional strategies for managing the feelings that come with those tasks. The techniques discussed here go beyond simply completing your to-do list; they aim to transform your approach to time management into a more positive and proactive experience. As you move forward, remember that effective time management is not just about clocks and calendars, but also about managing your mind and emotions as you navigate your daily responsibilities. In the next chapter, we will explore further strategies to enhance focus and productivity, building on the foundations laid in addressing the common pitfalls and anxieties associated with time management.

4

LEVERAGING TECHNOLOGY FOR ENHANCED FOCUS

As we live in the digital era, the seamless integration of technology into our daily lives brings a unique sense of hope and relief. This is especially true for those of us navigating the challenges of ADHD. It's like finding a compass in a dense forest; the right technological tools guide us and significantly enhance our journey through the complexities of time management. This chapter is dedicated to unraveling the digital threads that can weave a tapestry of structured, focused, and productive days for someone with ADHD, highlighting technology's unique benefits in this context.

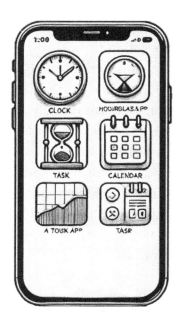

APPS THAT WORK: TIME MANAGEMENT IN THE DIGITAL AGE

In the vast ocean of applications, discovering the ones that act not just as a band-aid but as a potent remedy for ADHD-related time management challenges can be truly transformative. These apps are not just tools; they are lifelines that extend functionality, simplicity, and adaptability—qualities that resonate deeply with the needs of the ADHD community. They empower us and offer a hopeful path toward better time management, potentially transforming how we navigate our daily tasks and responsibilities and giving us a sense of control and confidence.

Overview of Beneficial Apps

Navigating through the App Store or Google Play can feel overwhelming with the myriad options available. However, some gems shine brightly for their effectiveness in catering specifically to the nuanced needs of individuals with ADHD. Apps like Trello, Asana, and Todoist stand out for their robust task management features. They allow you to segment large projects into manageable tasks, set deadlines, and update statuses on the go. For those who struggle with time perception, apps like Forest offer a creative solution by encouraging focus while discouraging phone use, helping you stay on task by growing virtual trees that flourish as you work.

Then there's Notion or Obsidian, versatile apps perfect for those who need to jot down every spark of an idea before it flutters away. They offer note-taking, organizing, task lists, and archiving, indispensable for keeping track of sprawling projects and thoughts. For reminders and scheduling, Google Keep and Microsoft To-Do provide straightforward, easy-to-use interfaces that help keep your day on track without clutter or complication.

Features That Make a Difference

The true power of these apps lies in their features that specifically address common ADHD challenges. The ability to sync across multiple devices is crucial. It ensures that whether you're on your phone, tablet, or computer, your tasks and schedules are always at your fingertips, updated in real time. This connectivity is vital for keeping up with the fast-paced, often chaotic life rhythms many with ADHD experience.

Another critical feature is intuitive design. Apps with user-friendly interfaces reduce the cognitive load, making them more accessible and less frustrating to use regularly. Such a design makes you feel less overwhelmed and more in control, enhancing your experience with these apps.

Integrating Apps Into Daily Life

Introducing these apps into your daily routine should enhance your productivity, not complicate it. Start by identifying specific time management areas in which you struggle, such as task completion, procrastination, or simply remembering appointments. Then, choose one or two apps that address these areas and slowly integrate them into your routine. For instance, if keeping track of multiple deadlines is challenging, an app like Todoist can help manage your projects with reminders and due dates.

It's important to give yourself time to adjust to these tools. Integrating technology effectively into your life isn't about overhauling your routines overnight but rather about making gradual changes that build toward significant improvements. Regularly assess how these apps affect your productivity and adjust as needed, either by tweaking your current tools or introducing new apps into your repertoire. Be prepared for potential challenges such as app compatibility issues or learning curves, and remember that seeking help from support resources or communities can be beneficial. Patience and persistence are essential in this journey, and every step forward is a step toward a more focused and productive life.

Harnessing the right digital tools can be a game-changer in managing ADHD's multifaceted challenges. As you explore these apps, remember that technology is here to serve you—to simplify your tasks, remind you of your commitments, and free up your mind for higher pursuits. Let these digital solutions be your ally in crafting a more focused, productive, and balanced life.

GAMIFICATION OF TIME MANAGEMENT TASKS

Transforming the way you approach daily tasks, especially when you have ADHD, can sometimes feel like trying to solve a complex puzzle with missing pieces. This is where the concept of gamification comes into play. Gamification is the application of typical elements of game playing (e.g., point scoring, competition with others, rules of play) to other areas of activity, typically as an online marketing technique to encourage engagement with a product or service. In the context of managing ADHD, it's a strategy that infuses the elements of game design into non-game environments, like your daily routines and tasks. Gamification taps into the natural desires for competition, achievement, and reward. For individuals with ADHD who may struggle with sustained motivation and engagement, this can be particularly effective in turning mundane or challenging tasks into engaging, even enjoyable, activities.

Imagine transforming your daily to-do list into a quest, where completing each task earns you points and badges or advances you to the next level. This method makes the process more fun and provides clear milestones and rewards that help maintain interest and motivation. For instance, consider the simple task of filing paperwork, which is often tedious. Setting up a point system where each file sorted earns you points, and reaching 100 points rewards you with a coffee break or a small treat, which makes the task more engaging. By gamifying this task, you're not just filing paperwork; you're earning rewards and achieving goals along the way.

Progress tracking is another integral element of gamification that resonates well with ADHD management. Visual progress bars or completion meters can provide immediate feedback that something has been accomplished, which is incredibly satisfying and motivating. This feedback helps build positive momentum, where each completed task propels you to enthusiastically tackle the next one. For example, using an app that tracks your progress on a project and visually represents how much you've completed can give you a tangible sense of achievement, encouraging you to keep going.

Tools and Platforms for Gamification

Several digital tools and platforms are designed with gamification in mind, specifically to enhance productivity and focus. Habitica is a tool that gamifies your daily life by turning all your tasks and goals into little monsters you must conquer. The more tasks you complete, the stronger your character becomes, allowing you to battle more enormous monsters—a fun and imaginative way to stay on track. Similarly, the Forest app uses the concept of planting a virtual tree that grows as you focus on your tasks. If you move away from your task, the tree withers, providing a visual stake in maintaining focus.

These apps make task management more engaging and weave in the critical elements of ADHD management—structure, consistency, and rewards. Integrating these apps into your daily routine can be as simple as setting up daily goals in the app each morning and checking them off as you complete them throughout the day. The key is consistency; the more you use these tools, the more effective they become in helping you build and maintain productive habits.

Balancing Fun and Functionality

While gamification can add fun and excitement to task management, it's crucial to maintain a balance to ensure it remains a productivity tool and not just a source of entertainment. One way to achieve this balance is by setting clear goals for what you need to accomplish and establishing rules for how you engage with the gamified system. For instance, you can only claim rewards if you complete a certain number of tasks or stick to your designated task times.

It's also important to periodically review the effectiveness of your gamification strategy. Ask yourself whether the game elements still serve their purpose in making task management more manageable and enjoyable or if they are becoming distractions themselves. If it's the latter, it might be time to adjust the rules, change the rewards, or try a different tool that suits your current needs better.

By carefully crafting a gamified system that is fun yet functional, you can transform your approach to daily tasks and projects. This makes day-to-day activities more enjoyable and enhances overall productivity, making it easier to navigate the challenges of ADHD with a renewed sense of motivation and engagement. Embrace these tools and strategies as part of your toolkit in managing time and tasks, and you may find that what once felt like a mundane or daunting part of your day becomes a source of triumph and enjoyment.

USING MIND MAPPING TOOLS FOR BETTER TASK ORGANIZATION

For someone with ADHD, the visual layout of a mind map can be beneficial, turning a jumble of thoughts and tasks into a clear visual diagram. Mind mapping allows you to capture thoughts, ideas, and tasks visually, which can be particularly beneficial if you find linear lists or traditional notes too restrictive or challenging to follow. This method offers a bird's-eye view of your project or task, making it easier to see connections, prioritize actions, and allocate your focus effectively. By mapping out tasks and ideas, you can visually track your project's components and status, which helps maintain focus and motivation as you see your progress reflected in the evolving map.

Benefits of Mind Mapping

The core advantage of mind mapping lies in its ability to break down complex information into a structured, visual format that is easy to understand and interact with. For individuals with ADHD, this is invaluable. It helps reduce the overwhelm by visually categorizing and prioritizing tasks, ideas, and projects. Additionally, mind maps can be dynamically adjusted as new ideas or tasks arise, which is often the case in the fluid, fast-paced thought processes characteristic of ADHD. The flexibility to expand and modify your map without losing coherence is crucial, allowing the mind map to evolve as your project or under-standing grows.

Choosing the Right Mind Mapping Tool

Selecting the right tool for mind mapping is crucial to ensure that the process enhances your productivity rather than adding to your cognitive load. The ideal tool should be intuitive, requiring minimal learning time so that you can focus more on the task than on learning the software. Look for tools that offer accessible drag-and-drop features, straightforward editing options, and the ability to insert images or links easily.

Flexibility is another critical feature; the tool should allow you to easily rearrange ideas and tasks as your project develops or your priorities change. Additionally, consider whether you need the ability to collaborate with others on your mind maps. If so, choose software that supports real-time collaboration and can sync across multiple devices, ensuring that all participants view the map's most up-to-date version.

Step-By-Step Guide to Creating Effective Mind Maps

Creating a practical mind map involves several key steps. Start with the central idea or project theme at the center of your map. Draw branches from this central node for each primary subtopic or task area related to your central idea. For example, if your project is to organize a community event, the main branches could include "venue," "publicity," "tickets," and "program."

From each of these branches, draw smaller branches to represent specific tasks or ideas related to each subtopic. Under "venue," you might have branches like "research options," "visit sites," and "book venue." Use keywords or short phrases rather than lengthy sentences to keep the map clear and easy to read. You can use different colors for different branches to enhance the visual separation of various sections of your project, which aids in mental categorization and recall.

As you add to your mind map, you may find new connections between different branches or realize that some tasks must be prioritized over others. Adjust the map as needed, moving branches or adding new nodes. This flexibility is one of the strengths of mind mapping, especially for ADHD, as it allows the map to be a dynamic, evolving representation of your thought process and project management.

Case Studies of Successful Mind Mapping

Real-life applications of mind mapping often highlight its effectiveness in enhancing clarity and organization, which is crucial for managing ADHD. Consider the case of Sarah, a freelance digital marketer who struggled to track multiple client projects. Using a mind mapping tool, Sarah could create separate maps for each project, with branches for each major task area, like content creation, SEO, and client feedback. This helped her keep her projects organized and made it easier to update clients on project progress, as she could quickly show them the current state of the mind map.

Another example is John, a high school teacher with ADHD who found lesson planning challenging due to his students' diverse needs and the complexity of the topics covered. John started using mind mapping to plan his lessons, with branches for each key topic and sub-branches for different teaching activities and resources. This approach allowed him to adapt his plans to better suit his students' needs, as he could easily see where more attention was needed or where additional resources could be beneficial.

These examples underscore how mind mapping can transform the management of complex tasks and projects into a more manageable, less overwhelming process. By visually organizing your thoughts and tasks, you can navigate the challenges of ADHD with greater ease, ensuring that your energy is spent on practical task completion rather than struggling with organization and prioritization. As you continue exploring and utilizing mind mapping, you may find that what once seemed like impossible projects become a series of well-structured tasks you can confidently manage and execute.

PRODUCTIVITY BOOSTERS: FROM POMODORO TO TIME BLOCKING

In the bustling rhythm of life, especially when juggling the added layers of ADHD, finding effective ways to manage time isn't just helpful—it's essential. Two tried-and-true methods that stand out for their adaptability and effectiveness are the Pomodoro Technique and time blocking. Both strategies offer structured ways to organize your tasks but also bring much-needed clarity and focus, which can often be elusive when your mind manages a million thoughts simultaneously.

However, traditional Pomodoro intervals are not a one-size-fits-all solution, especially for ADHD minds that might need more frequent breaks or shorter focus periods. Adapting the length of the Pomodoro intervals can be incredibly helpful. For instance, working for 15 minutes and breaking for 5 minutes might work better for you. The key is experimenting with different intervals to find a rhythm that keeps you productive but not drained.

Time blocking is another technique that involves dividing your day into blocks of time, each dedicated to accomplishing a specific task or group of functions. This method helps by visually mapping out your day in advance, which can reduce anxiety and indecision about what to do, common issues for those with ADHD. By seeing your day planned out, you can mentally prepare for what's coming and transition more smoothly from one activity to the next.

To tailor time blocking for ADHD, incorporating more frequent breaks and varying the length of time blocks according to the nature of the task or your current mental state can be effective. For instance, high-focus tasks might be scheduled during peak mental alertness times, while more mundane tasks can be placed in blocks where your energy dips.

Tools to Support These Techniques

Incorporating digital tools that support these techniques can further enhance their effectiveness. Apps like Focus Keeper or Pomodone App integrate the Pomodoro Technique with task management features, allowing you to customize the length of focus periods and breaks to suit your needs. They also provide visual and auditory cues to guide you through your Pomodoros, helping keep you on track.

Calendar apps like Google Calendar or Outlook are invaluable for time blocking. They allow you to color-code different blocks of time according to the type of activity, making your schedule easy to scan and understand at a glance. Adding alerts before transitions can also help manage the switch between tasks, a standard stumbling block for many with ADHD.

Success Stories

Many individuals with ADHD have found these techniques transformative. For instance, a graphic designer named Eliza shares how adapting the Pomodoro Technique allowed her to manage her freelance projects more effectively. By adjusting the work intervals to 20 minutes, she could maintain focus without feeling over-whelmed, dramatically increasing her productivity and reducing her work-related stress.

Similarly, a software developer named Raj found that time blocking enabled him to manage his varied responsibilities, from coding to meetings, without the usual chaos. By planning his day in distinct blocks and using a digital calendar to remind him of transitions, he could give each task his full attention, leading to higher quality work and less mental fatigue.

With their adaptability and focus on managing energy and atten-tion, these techniques offer practical solutions for enhancing productivity and focus in individuals with ADHD. By experi-menting with and adjusting these methods, you can find a system that works uniquely for you, turning potential daily struggles into opportunities for success and satisfaction.

As we wrap up this exploration of productivity boosters, remember the key takeaway: structured time management tech-niques like Pomodoro and time blocking can be highly effective, especially when adapted to meet the unique needs of the ADHD mind. By utilizing supportive digital tools and learning from the experiences of others who share similar challenges, you can craft a personalized approach to productivity that respects your mental rhythms and enhances your daily efficiency.

In the next chapter, we will dive into strategies that help manage time and enhance the overall quality of life, ensuring that you're productive and living well with ADHD.

5

EMOTIONAL INSIGHTS AND SUPPORT SYSTEMS

Imagine standing at the edge of a high dive at a pool, the water shimmering invitingly below. There's a moment of hesitation, a flutter of anxiety—do you have what it takes to leap? For adults with ADHD, every task can sometimes feel like standing on that high dive. The anticipation of beginning can often 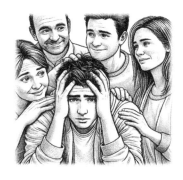 be the most challenging part, muddied by anxiety and fraught with a fear of failure.

This chapter is dedicated to unpacking that moment on the edge, transforming it from a point of paralysis to one of empowered action. Here, we dive into managing task-related anxiety, a common but surmountable challenge that can significantly impact your ability to engage with and complete tasks efficiently.

UNDERSTANDING AND MANAGING TASK-RELATED ANXIETY

Task-related anxiety in individuals with ADHD can often be traced back to specific triggers. Identifying these triggers is the first step toward managing them effectively. Common sources of stress might include a daunting project scope, fear of failure, or even the pressure of meeting high expectations. These triggers can induce a fight-or-flight response that is counterproductive to completing the task at hand.

To identify your personal anxiety triggers, start by observing patterns in your reactions to different tasks. Keep a journal where you note instances of anxiety, detailing the task, the time, and the specific aspects that seem to contribute to your stress. This self-monitoring can highlight recurring themes or situations that particularly heighten your anxiety. For instance, you might find that tasks requiring sustained attention cause more anxiety than brief and varied tasks. This suggests that breaking tasks into smaller, more manageable chunks could alleviate some of the stress.

Cognitive Behavioral Technique

Once you've identified your triggers, cognitive behavioral techniques can be incredibly effective in managing task-related anxiety. These techniques involve identifying negative, often irrational thoughts that fuel your anxiety and systematically challenging them to reshape your thinking patterns. It's about recognizing when you're thinking negatively and finding evidence to prove those thoughts wrong.

For example, if you usually think, "I'm going to mess this up," challenge this thought with proof of past successes or by examining the realistic outcomes of making a mistake, which is often less catastrophic than your anxiety would have you believe.

Practicing these techniques consistently can fundamentally alter how you perceive and react to tasks, reducing anxiety and improving your approach to work and deadlines. Engaging with a cognitive-behavioral therapist can provide further personalized strategies and support, but many resources, such as workbooks and online courses, can also guide you through this process independently.

Relaxation Strategies

With cognitive behavioral techniques, relaxation strategies can play a crucial role in managing anxiety. Techniques such as deep breathing, progressive muscle relaxation, and guided imagery can be used to calm your mind and body, particularly before and during task execution. For deep breathing, focus on taking slow, deep breaths, inhaling through your nose, and exhaling through your mouth, which can help reduce the physical symptoms of anxiety like rapid heartbeat or sweating. And as mentioned in a previous chapter, progressive muscle relaxation involves tensing and then relaxing different muscle groups in your body can help release the physical tension associated with anxiety.

Building a Pre-task Routine

Creating a calming pre-task routine can also significantly ease task-related anxiety. This routine should include activities that help you transition into a focused and calm state. For example, you might spend a few minutes meditating, listening to soothing music, or doing a brief physical activity like stretching or walking. Incorporate one or more of the relaxation strategies you've found effective into this routine. The consistency of a pre-task routine prepares your body and mind for the work ahead and signals that it's time to focus, helping to create a psychological barrier between your anxious thoughts and the task at hand.

Interactive Element: Anxiety Management Exercise

To put these strategies into practice, try the following exercise: Next time you face a task that triggers anxiety, pause and write down the specific thoughts contributing to your stress. Challenge these thoughts with evidence or alternative outcomes, use a brief relaxation technique like deep breathing or progressive muscle relaxation, and proceed with your pre-task routine. Reflect on this process in your journal, noting any changes in your anxiety levels or task engagement. This reflective practice can enhance your understanding of which strategies are most effective for you and how best to implement them in your daily life.

By understanding and addressing task-related anxiety with these targeted strategies, you can transform your approach to tasks from dread and avoidance to engagement and accomplishment. This transformation is empowering, as it shifts the goal from eliminating anxiety to managing it so that it no longer controls your actions or hinders your productivity. With practice and persistence, you can turn anxiety from a stumbling block into a stepping stone, paving the way for more focused, efficient, and successful task completion. This empowerment is a testament to your resilience and determination, inspiring you to take on tasks with renewed vigor and confidence.

THE ROLE OF EMOTIONAL SUPPORT IN ADHD TIME MANAGEMENT

Navigating the complexities of ADHD often requires more than just personal willpower and self-management strategies; it demands a supportive network that understands, encourages, and aids in your journey toward better time management. Emotional support is not just a pillar but a lifeline that can uplift your spirits, clarify your thoughts, and keep you anchored during turbulent times. This support, whether from friends, family, or therapists, is a testament to your value and the understanding that you are not alone in your struggles with ADHD. It's a reminder that there are people who care about you and are ready to stand by you in your journey.

When you consider the impact of emotional support, it's essential to recognize that ADHD often brings with it feelings of isolation or misunderstanding. A supportive relationship, therefore, serves as a bridge between these feelings and the world around you, offering a sense of connection and understanding that can be profoundly reassuring. For instance, friends and family who acknowledge your struggles without judgment can boost your morale and motivate you to persevere through challenging tasks. On the other hand, therapists or coaches specializing in ADHD can offer professional insights that refine your approach to time management, providing tailored strategies that align with your unique cognitive patterns and lifestyle needs.

Each type of supportive relationship contributes differently to your management of ADHD. Friends may offer a listening ear or a distraction when needed, helping you manage stress and recharge your mental batteries. Family members might assist in more practical ways, such as reminding you of appointments or helping maintain a routine, easing daily pressures. Professional support, such as from therapists or ADHD coaches, brings a structured approach to tackling ADHD-related challenges, focusing on developing coping mechanisms that enhance time management skills and overall productivity.

Strategies for Seeking Support

Building and maintaining these supportive relationships requires thoughtful communication and mutual understanding. Expressing your needs clearly and effectively is crucial and sometimes daunting. Start by identifying what type of support you find most helpful. Do you need someone to help you track tasks or discuss your frustrations and achievements? Once you understand your needs, communicate them openly with your potential support network. Be specific about what helps and doesn't, and be open to hearing their thoughts on how they can best support you.

For instance, you might explain to a family member that it helps when they check in with you about your daily tasks, or you might ask a friend to be your accountability partner in a project. In professional settings, such as with a therapist or coach, setting clear goals for what you wish to achieve from the sessions can lead to more targeted and practical support.

Engaging in consistent dialogue about your progress, struggles, and strategies for managing ADHD fosters a more in-depth understanding between you and your supporters, which can enhance the quality of support you receive. Additionally, being open to feedback and willing to adjust your approaches based on constructive criticism can lead to improved strategies and stronger supportive relationships.

Support Groups and Communities

Beyond individual relationships, participating in support groups and online communities for individuals with ADHD can offer additional layers of understanding and camaraderie. These groups provide a platform to share experiences, challenges, and successes with others navigating similar paths. The collective wisdom found in these groups can be precious, offering diverse perspectives and coping strategies that might not be available in your immediate environment.

Online forums, social media groups, and local meet-ups can serve as access points to these communities. Engaging with these groups can help you feel less isolated in your struggles and more empowered to manage your challenges effectively. Many members find comfort and motivation in sharing their journey with others who understand the intricacies of living with ADHD.

For example, participating in a weekly online forum where members share their time management successes and setbacks could provide you with new insights and methods to try in your own life. Additionally, many of these groups often compile resources, such as lists of ADHD-friendly tools or professional services, which can be extremely useful.

By understanding the critical role of emotional support in managing ADHD and actively engaging in supportive relationships and communities, you can enhance your ability to manage time and tasks more effectively. This support network provides practical help and emotional reassurance and enriches your journey toward personal and professional fulfillment, making the path less daunting and more connected.

CREATING A SUPPORTIVE ENVIRONMENT AT HOME AND WORK

In your quest to master time management with ADHD, the spaces where you live, work, and play are pivotal roles. These environments can either serve as sanctuaries that bolster your focus and productivity or battlegrounds cluttered with distractions that sap your energy and disrupt your flow. Optimizing these physical spaces is not just about organization; it's about creating an atmosphere that actively supports your efforts to manage time and reduces stress.

Let's start with organizing your living and working spaces. Clutter is often the enemy of focus, particularly for the ADHD mind, which can be easily sidetracked. A clean, well-organized environment can significantly affect your ability to concentrate and stay on task. Begin by decluttering your primary workspaces. This doesn't mean you need a stark, sterile environment where everything has a place and unnecessary distractions are minimized. Use organizational tools like shelves, bins, and digital tools to keep necessary items within reach but out of the immediate line of sight when not in use. For paperwork, consider a filing system that's easy to maintain and regularly set aside time to keep this system organized.

Moreover, consider the layout of your space. Position your desk or main work area so that it faces away from high-traffic areas or windows that might offer too much distraction. Use natural light to your advantage; it's been shown to boost mood and productivity. For those times when focus is paramount, have items on hand that help block out distractions—noise-canceling headphones can be invaluable in a noisy environment. Room dividers can help create a more secluded space if needed.

Creating a supportive emotional climate is equally crucial. This includes managing relationships with those you share these spaces with, be it family at home or colleagues at work. Open communication about your ADHD and how it impacts your work can help others understand your needs and contribute to a more supportive environment. Discuss how unavoidable interruptions might disrupt your flow more than they realize, and work together to develop solutions that benefit everyone. For instance, setting specific 'do not disturb' times when you need to focus intensely can help others know when to avoid interrupting you and when it's a better time to connect.

Negotiating accommodations at work or school is another strategy that can significantly impact your ability to manage time effectively. Many workplaces and educational institutions are becoming more aware of the needs associated with ADHD, and reasonable accommodations can often be made if approached correctly. Start by understanding what changes would most benefit your productivity —whether it's flexibility in your schedule to allow for work during peak focus times or having access to a quiet workspace away from the usual hustle and bustle. When you approach your employer or educational advisor, be clear and specific about what accommodations you need and why. It's also helpful to suggest practical solutions that might not require significant changes on their part. For example, you can request approval to use noise-canceling headphones if the office environment is particularly loud or request written summaries of meetings to ensure you can fully process the information discussed.

Finally, involving others in finding solutions to enhance productivity can foster a more profound understanding and stronger cooperation. At home, this might mean working with family members to establish routines that reduce morning chaos or setting up shared calendars so everyone knows each other's schedules and can plan accordingly. This could involve collaborating with colleagues to set up a workflow or project management system that keeps everyone better organized and on track. Involving others helps them understand your challenges and allows them to contribute to creating an environment where everyone can thrive.

By optimizing your physical and emotional environment, you can create spaces that support your ADHD and enhance your overall productivity and well-being. Whether through better organization, strategic accommodations, or cooperative problem-solving, each adjustment brings you closer to a lifestyle where time management becomes less of a struggle and more of a successful endeavor.

SELF-MOTIVATION TECHNIQUES THAT REALLY WORK FOR ADHD

Understanding the unique interplay between ADHD and motivation reveals why traditional motivational strategies often fall short for those with ADHD. Your experience may fluctuate dramatically —some days, you're driven and can tackle any challenge enthusiastically; other days, minor tasks seem impossible. This inconsistency isn't a failure of willpower but rather a characteristic of how ADHD affects energy levels and interest. Recognizing this pattern is crucial because it helps frame your approach to self-motivation to accommodate these fluctuations instead of fighting against them.

Developing effective reward systems can significantly enhance your motivation, especially when tailored to meet your personal preferences and the realities of living with ADHD. The key is to identify rewards that genuinely resonate with you and are immediately gratifying enough to overcome the lure of distraction. For instance, if you complete a morning of focused work, you might reward yourself with a favorite coffee or a short episode of a show you enjoy. These rewards should be easy to deliver and directly tied to completing a task to reinforce the behavior. It's also helpful to vary the rewards to prevent them from becoming stale and losing their motivational power.

Setting up these reward systems begins with simply listing tasks and corresponding rewards. Keep this list visible in your workspace to remind you what you can look forward to by staying focused. Additionally, involve someone you trust to help you manage this system—having an accountability partner can enhance the effectiveness of the rewards, providing an additional layer of motivation through social reinforcement. This partner can help you celebrate when you claim a reward, making the achievement feel even more substantial.

Visualizing success is another potent technique that can bolster your motivation. This practice involves creating a vivid mental image of the outcome you desire, engaging as many senses as possible to enhance the realism of the visualization. For instance, if your goal is to complete a significant project, spend a few minutes each day picturing yourself putting the final touches on the project, imagining the sense of satisfaction and relief you will feel. Visualizing the positive feedback you might receive can also amplify your emotional investment in the tasks necessary to achieve that outcome.

The process of visualization not only increases your emotional engagement with your goals but primes your brain to recognize and pursue paths that will lead to the desired outcome, effectively turning your visualizations into a roadmap for success. Regular practice can make these mental images a motivational anchor, helping you maintain focus on your goals, especially during periods of low interest or energy.

Maintaining motivation over the long term requires continual adjustment and celebration of milestones. Set smaller, interim goals as steps toward your larger objectives. Celebrating these minor victories can provide ongoing motivation and a sense of progress, which is especially important in maintaining your drive during more extended projects. For instance, if you're working on a significant report, you might set a goal to complete each section before a specific date and treat yourself to something enjoyable as a reward for meeting each deadline.

Regularly reviewing and revisiting your goals and strategies is also crucial. This helps you stay aligned with your changing priorities and circumstances and fine-tune your approach based on what has been effective or not. Schedule a monthly review session where you assess your progress, reflect on what's working and what isn't, and adjust your goals and motivational strategies accordingly. This process ensures that your approach to motivation evolves along with your personal and professional growth, keeping your strategy fresh and closely aligned with your current needs and aspirations.

By embracing these self-motivation techniques and integrating them into your daily life, you can create a sustainable approach that respects the unique challenges of ADHD and harnesses your personal strengths. Whether through tailored reward systems, vivid visualizations of success, or strategic celebrations of progress, these techniques provide a framework for consistently moving forward, even in the face of ADHD's inherent fluctuations in energy and interest. As you continue to apply and adjust these strategies, they become not just tools for achieving specific goals but fundamental components of a fulfilling, motivated lifestyle.

DEALING WITH SETBACKS: A RESILIENT APPROACH TO TIME MANAGEMENT

Setbacks are an inevitable part of managing time, especially when you're navigating the complexities of ADHD. It's natural to feel as though every missed deadline or overlooked task is a step back, but the truth is, these moments are opportunities. Normalizing the experience of setbacks in your journey of time management is crucial. Understanding that these are not failures but part of the learning process can significantly reduce the self-judgment that often accompanies such moments. Acknowledging your feelings about these setbacks and viewing them through a lens of growth and understanding is essential.

When encountering a setback, the first reaction might be frustration or disappointment, which is entirely valid. However, shifting your perspective to see these situations as chances to learn can transform your approach to managing time. This mindset encourages a detailed examination of what went awry and why. Was the planning phase inadequate? Did unexpected challenges arise? Reflecting on these questions can provide valuable insights into your time management strategies and help refine them for future tasks.

For instance, if you consistently underestimate the time needed for specific tasks, this realization can lead you to adjust your future estimates and planning strategies, potentially leading to more realistic scheduling and less stress about time constraints. This continuous learning process can significantly enhance your ability to manage time effectively, turning what might feel like a step back into a proactive stride forward.

Resilience-Building Strategies

Building resilience against setbacks involves developing tools and strategies that help you recover and move forward. One particularly effective tool is a setback journal. This can be a dedicated notebook or digital document where you record details about each setback, what you think caused it, how it made you feel, and what steps you took to overcome it. Regularly reviewing this journal can offer insights into patterns that may not be obvious and help you develop strategies to avoid similar issues in the future.

Another critical aspect of building resilience is setting small, achievable goals leading to larger objectives. This approach makes tasks seem less daunting and provides frequent opportunities for success. Each small victory builds your confidence and reinforces your ability to manage your time effectively, even in the face of challenges. Over time, this builds a resilience that makes setbacks less intimidating and more manageable.

Support Systems for Recovery

The role of support systems in navigating setbacks cannot be overstated. Whether it's family, friends, or colleagues, having people who understand your challenges and support your efforts can significantly affect how you recover from setbacks. These support systems provide emotional reassurance, practical help, and perspectives that might not be apparent when facing challenges alone.

For example, a family member might help you brainstorm solutions to a time management problem, or a colleague could share strategies that have worked for them in similar situations. Sometimes, talking through your frustrations and successes with someone can be valuable. This support can bolster your morale and motivate you to tackle the next challenge.

Consider seeking formal support mechanisms in professional or educational settings as well. This might include working with a counselor, joining a support group for individuals with ADHD, or engaging with a professional organizer or coach specializing in time management. These resources can provide specialized strategies and support tailored to your specific needs, enhancing your ability to manage time effectively despite setbacks.

By embracing these strategies and understanding the value of setbacks as learning opportunities, you can develop a resilient approach to time management that accommodates the ups and downs of life with ADHD. This resilience improves your ability to handle setbacks and enhances your confidence and competence in managing time, turning potential stumbling blocks into stepping stones for success.

In wrapping up this chapter, remember that setbacks are not roadblocks on your path to effective time management but rather signposts that offer direction and guidance. Each challenge provides unique insights into your personal time management style and offers opportunities to refine your strategies and strengthen your skills. As we transition into the next chapter, we carry forward the resilience and learning cultivated here, ready to explore advanced techniques that build on these foundational skills.

MAKE A DIFFERENCE WITH YOUR REVIEW AND UNLOCK THE POWER OF GENEROSITY

"Money can't buy happiness, but giving it away can."

— FREDDIE MERCURY

People who give without expectation live longer, happier lives and make more money. So if we've got a shot at that during our time together, darn it, I'm gonna try.

To make that happen, I have a question for you...

Would you help someone you've never met, even if you never got credit for it?

Who is this person you ask? They are like you. Or, at least, like you used to be. Less experienced, wanting to make a difference, and needing help, but not sure where to look.

Our mission is to make time management strategies for adults with ADHD accessible to everyone. Everything I do stems from that mission. And, the only way for me to accomplish that mission is by reaching...well...everyone.

This is where you come in. Most people do, in fact, judge a book by its cover (and its reviews). So here's my ask on behalf of a struggling adult with ADHD you've never met:

Please help that person by leaving this book a review.

Your gift costs no money and less than 60 seconds to make real, but can change a fellow reader's life forever. Your review could help…

- one more adult find focus in their daily life.
- one more person reduce their stress and anxiety.
- one more reader balance their work and personal life.
- one more individual gain confidence in managing their time.
- one more dream come true.

To get that 'feel good' feeling and help this person for real, all you have to do is...and it takes less than 60 seconds...leave a review.

Simply scan the QR code or visit the link below to leave your review on Amazon:
www.adhdtimemgmtreview.com

If you feel good about helping a faceless reader, you are my kind of person. Welcome to the club. You're one of us.

I'm that much more excited to help you achieve your goals faster, easier, and more effectively than you can possibly imagine. You'll love the strategies I'm about to share in the coming chapters.

Thank you from the bottom of my heart. Now, back to our regularly scheduled program.

Your biggest fan,

Noelle Walker

PS - Fun fact: If you provide something of value to another person, it makes you more valuable to them. If you'd like goodwill straight from another reader - and you believe this book will help them - send this book their way.

6

ADVANCED STRATEGIES FOR LONG-TERM PLANNING

Imagine setting sail on a vast ocean, navigating toward a horizon that stretches endlessly before you. Planning for the long term with ADHD can often feel like charting a course through such boundless waters—daunting, yes, but also filled with potential for discovery and achievement. As you steer 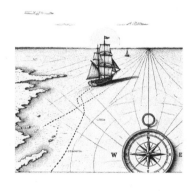 through these waters, your strategies can make the difference between drifting aimlessly and reaching exciting new destinations. This chapter is your compass, designed to help you map out your long-term goals with clarity and purpose, ensuring that the journey ahead is not just navigated but enjoyed.

MASTERING LONG-TERM GOAL SETTING WITH ADHD

Understanding Long-Term Goals

Long-term goals are not just markers of what you hope to achieve; they are lighthouses guiding you through the foggy days when ADHD symptoms feel overwhelming. For individuals with ADHD, the challenge often lies in the abstract nature of such goals, which can seem distant and disconnected from daily realities. However, recognizing the importance of these goals in your personal and professional growth is the first step. They provide a clear direction and motivation, helping you focus on what truly matters, even when distractions abound.

Setting long-term goals is crucial because it aligns your shorter-term actions and decisions with your larger aspirations. Whether advancing in your career, improving your health, or forging more robust relationships, each goal is a stepping stone toward a more prosperous, more fulfilling life. However, setting these goals also needs to account for the unique challenges posed by ADHD, including the tendency for time blindness, difficulty in maintaining focus over extended periods, and the need for immediate gratification.

SMART Goals for ADHD

The SMART framework can be a powerful tool for making long-term goals tangible and achievable. Conceived initially to set objectives in management settings, SMART stands for Specific, Measurable, Achievable, Relevant, and Time-bound. Adapting this framework to suit the needs of someone with ADHD involves emphasizing flexibility and clear, achievable milestones.

SMART Goal Setting

S	Specific: Define a clear, specific goal.
M	Measurable: Make sure you can track progress.
A	Attainable: Create a goal that is realistic.
R	Relevant: Ensure your goal aligns with the organization.
T	Time-bound: Assign a target date to keep accountable.

For example, a goal like "Improve health" is too vague and can be overwhelming. Reframing it as "Walk 30 minutes a day, 5 days a week, to improve cardiovascular health within the next 6 months" makes it Specific, Measurable (tracking daily walks), Achievable (a reasonable time frame), Relevant (directly impacting health), and Time-bound (6 months). This clarity breaks down the goal into daily actions that are easier to manage and keep track of, which is particularly helpful when you struggle to focus on long-term outcomes.

Visual Goal-Setting Techniques

Visual tools can bring your goals to life, making them vivid and engaging. Vision boards, for instance, are a creative way to visually represent your goals using images, quotes, and symbols that resonate with your aspirations. Placing this board in a spot where you see it daily can serve as a constant reminder and source of motivation.

Mind maps are another visual technique for articulating and organizing goals. Starting with a central idea, you can branch out into specific tasks and objectives, creating a visual "map" of your path toward each goal. This method helps maintain focus and identify the connections between various goals and the steps needed to achieve them.

Ongoing Goal Adjustment

The fluid nature of life, especially with ADHD, means that your long-term goals will need regular review and adjustment. As you encounter new experiences, learn more about yourself, and navigate changes in your personal and professional life, your goals must evolve to reflect your current reality. This ongoing adjustment is not about straying from your path but refining it to ensure it remains aligned with your growth and aspirations.

Setting regular intervals for reviewing your goals, perhaps every 3 to 6 months, allows you to assess your progress, reflect on what's working or not, and make necessary adjustments. This process is not about veering off course, but about ensuring that your path continues to reflect your evolving growth and aspirations.

Interactive Element: Goal Mapping Exercise

To apply these concepts, try the following exercise:

1. **Create a Goal Map:** Using a large piece of paper or a digital tool, draw a central circle and write a long-term goal you wish to achieve.
2. **Branch Out:** Draw lines from the central circle to smaller circles, each representing specific actions or smaller goals that contribute to your main goal.
3. **Assign Time Frames:** Next to each action or smaller goal, write down a realistic time frame for achieving it.

4. **Visualize and Adjust:** Place your goal map somewhere you can see it daily. Use it to track your progress and make adjustments as needed.

This visual and interactive approach helps clarify and organize goals and integrate them into daily life, making each step toward them feel more deliberate and attainable.

As you continue to navigate through the complexities of setting and achieving long-term goals with ADHD, remember that each goal you set is not just a destination to be reached but a commitment to embark on a journey of personal growth and discovery. With the right strategies, these goals can transform from daunting tasks to exciting opportunities, each step bringing you closer to the person you aspire to become.

BREAKING DOWN LARGE PROJECTS INTO MANAGEABLE STEPS

When tackling a large project, the sheer magnitude of what needs to be done can feel overwhelming, especially when ADHD is in the mix. However, just as breaking down your daily tasks into smaller, manageable pieces has proven effective, the same approach can be applied to large projects. By deconstructing the project into smaller, achievable components, you can reduce the intimidation factor and create a series of steps that align with how your brain functions best—quick wins and shorter tasks that provide immediate satisfaction and a clear sense of progress. This not only empowers you with control over the project but also turns a daunting task into a series of manageable actions.

Traditional project management involves planning, executing, and monitoring activities to achieve specific goals. Yet, for individuals with ADHD, these conventional methods often require adaptation to better fit the way you naturally work. Frequent shifts in focus and the need for immediate gratification are typical in ADHD, and by customizing project management strategies to accommodate these tendencies, you can handle even the most complex projects with greater ease and effectiveness. Breaking down large tasks into smaller chunks isn't just a helpful tactic—it's a powerful tool that can turn potential obstacles into stepping stones toward success.

Iterative processes, which involve completing a project in small sections called iterations, are particularly effective. Each iteration delivers a part of the project's overall functionality and is planned and executed quickly, providing regular feedback and a sense of accomplishment that keeps motivation high. Frequent reviews at the end of each iteration allow for adjustments based on what's working and what's not, ensuring that the project remains aligned with your goals and adapts to any changes in your circumstances or priorities.

Task Segmentation Techniques

Breaking down a large project into smaller tasks is a critical strategy. Begin by mapping out the entire project to understand all the components involved. Then, break these components into tasks that can be completed in a few hours or a day. For example, if your project is to launch a personal blog, you can start by listing tasks such as choosing a blog platform, designing the blog, writing initial content, and promoting the blog. Each of these tasks can then be broken down further—choosing a blog platform involves researching different options, comparing features and pricing, and selecting the platform that best suits your needs. Designing the blog includes choosing a template or theme, customizing the design, and setting up essential pages like Home, About, and Contact. Writing initial content can be broken down into brainstorming blog post ideas, writing and editing the first few posts, and planning a content schedule. Finally, promoting the blog involves creating social media accounts, developing a promotion strategy, and engaging with potential readers by sharing your posts across various platforms.

This segmentation makes the tasks seem less daunting and allows you to approach the project with clear, focused steps. It's essential to prioritize these tasks based on their importance and deadlines. Use color-coding or tags to mark crucial and urgent tasks, ensuring they are addressed first. This visual prioritization helps quickly assess what needs your attention most, reducing the time spent deciding what to work on each day.

Utilizing Project Management Tools

Project management tools can be incredibly beneficial for keeping track of these tasks, especially ones that offer features tailored to the needs of someone with ADHD. Tools like Asana, Trello, or Monday.com allow you to create visual project boards where tasks can be organized by stages, priority, or any other criteria that make sense for your project. Features like reminders, due dates, and the ability to rearrange tasks easily are beneficial. These tools often support integrating other applications you might use, like calendars or communication tools, helping to keep all your project information in one accessible place.

For instance, you can set up a board for your community event project with columns for each central task area—venue, volunteers, promotions, and day-of logistics. As you complete tasks, move them to a "done" column, giving you a visual representation of your progress. Set reminders for tasks as their deadlines approach, ensuring nothing gets overlooked in the hustle of daily activities.

Real-Life Examples

Let's consider the example of Alex, a marketing consultant with ADHD tasked with leading an extensive, multi-month campaign for a new product launch. Initially overwhelmed by the scale of the project, Alex began by breaking down the campaign into phases such as research, planning, execution, and review. He used a digital project management tool to create a board for each phase, detailing the tasks and assigning deadlines and priorities. Alex managed the project successfully by focusing on completing one board at a time and using the tool's reminder features to stay on track, delivering results that exceeded his client's expectations.

Another case is that of Sarah, a freelance writer who decided to write a book. Faced with the daunting task of writing hundreds of pages, she broke the project down into chapters and then further into sections. Sarah used a simple project management app to track her progress on each section, set daily word count goals, and keep notes on her research. The app's ability to rearrange tasks easily was beneficial when she needed to shift her focus between different sections based on her research findings and creative flow.

These examples illustrate how large projects can be managed effectively with the right strategies and tools, turning potential overwhelm into structured progress. By breaking projects into manageable steps, utilizing supportive tools, and adapting project management principles to fit your working style, you can tackle large projects with confidence and success, turning them from sources of stress into opportunities for accomplishment and growth.

TIME MANAGEMENT FOR MAJOR LIFE EVENTS

Navigating major life events such as moving house, getting married, or starting a new job poses significant challenges in time management, particularly for individuals with ADHD. These events are not just mere changes; they are profound transitions that demand extensive planning, energy, and a high level of organization—elements that can often be overwhelming if ADHD is in the mix. The ADHD brain may grapple with these large-scale projects due to the need for detailed planning and prolonged focus, leading to heightened stress and anxiety during such periods.

The key to managing these life-changing events is early and thorough preparation. Building a detailed checklist is a foundational step in this preparation process. For instance, if you are planning a wedding, your checklist might include booking the venue, selecting a caterer, sending out invitations, and arranging transportation—all mapped out with specific deadlines. This checklist acts as a roadmap, guiding you through the myriad of tasks and helping ensure that nothing is overlooked. Each item checked off provides a slight sense of accomplishment and relief, reducing the overall stress associated with the event.

Using digital apps specifically designed for event planning can also significantly ease the management of these tasks. Apps like Trello or Asana allow you to create task lists, set reminders, and even share these tasks with others who might be helping you. For a house move, you could set up a board with lists for packing, utility transfers, and necessary purchases. Each task can be assigned a deadline, and the app can send reminders to your phone or email, helping keep everything on track. This digital approach helps manage the sheer volume of tasks. It maintains a clear overview of progress, which can be especially helpful when dealing with

ADHD-related challenges like forgetfulness or time misperception.

The importance of emotional and practical support during these transitions cannot be overstated. Major life events can be emotionally draining, making the ADHD symptoms more pronounced. This is where support from friends, family, or professionals can play a crucial role. Emotional support involves having people who understand the stresses associated with your ADHD and are there to offer encouragement and a listening ear. On the other hand, practical support involves hands-on help with the tasks at hand. For example, friends can help pack boxes for a move, or family members can assist in running errands for a wedding. Organizing this support effectively means being clear about what kind of help you need and communicating these needs to your support network. Let them know specific tasks you need help with, and don't hesitate to delegate.

Engaging in reflective practices after the event has concluded provides valuable insights that can improve future event planning and personal growth. This reflection involves looking back at what strategies worked, what didn't, and how ADHD played a role in the management of the event. Keeping a journal where you can jot down these reflections soon after the event can be particularly useful. You should note that breaking tasks down into smaller steps helped manage feelings of overwhelm or that specific tasks took longer than expected and required more time. These reflections provide a chance to pat yourself on the back for the successes and help you tweak your strategies for future events, making each major life event easier to manage than the last.

This approach to handling major life events with ADHD—through early planning with detailed checklists, leveraging technology, organizing support, and reflective practices—transforms daunting tasks into more manageable steps. It ensures you navigate these events more smoothly and builds skills and strategies that enhance your overall ability to manage time and projects effectively. As you move forward, each event becomes not just an occasion to celebrate or a challenge to overcome but also a learning experience, enriching your journey toward mastering ADHD and leading a fulfilling life.

ANTICIPATING AND PLANNING FOR ADHD TIME MANAGEMENT CHALLENGES

When managing long-term projects or goals, anticipating and planning for potential pitfalls can significantly enhance your ability to navigate them smoothly. ADHD brings its own set of challenges, such as the frequent underestimation of time required for tasks or the allure of new interests that can distract from current commitments. Understanding and preparing for these tendencies can prevent many common obstacles from derailing your progress.

Identifying potential pitfalls begins with a thorough self-assessment and reflection on past experiences. Consider times when you need to pay more attention to the duration of a project or be sidetracked by new ideas. These reflections help pinpoint specific patterns in your behavior and decision-making processes that could pose challenges in future planning. For instance, if you notice a recurring theme of distraction when engaging in multistep tasks, this insight allows you to strategize effectively against similar future disruptions.

Implementing preventative strategies is crucial in mitigating these identified risks. Setting interim deadlines is a practical approach to ensuring continuous progress and avoiding last-minute rushes, which are common in individuals with ADHD. These deadlines should be realistic, providing enough time to accommodate the hurdles without causing undue stress. External accountability, such as regular check-ins with a mentor or a peer group, can also significantly keep you on track. These accountability measures provide motivation and a platform for receiving constructive feedback, enabling adjustments before minor issues escalate into more critical problems.

Flexibility in planning is another critical element in managing long-term projects with ADHD. The variable nature of ADHD symptoms means that on some days, productivity might be high, while on others, it might wane significantly. Building flexibility into your plans allows you to capitalize on high-energy days and adjust for those times when focus is more challenging to maintain. This might involve having a buffer period for tasks or setting adjustable priorities that can shift depending on your daily state of mind and external circumstances. Such adaptability in planning acknowledges the ebb and flow of your capabilities and reduces the pressure to perform consistently, which is often unrealistic for someone managing ADHD.

Maintaining motivation over extended periods is another challenge, especially when the rewards or outcomes of your efforts take time. To keep your spirits high, integrate regular celebrations of small successes along the way. Recognizing and rewarding yourself for minor achievements helps sustain motivation and reinforces your commitment to the larger goal. Additionally, revisiting the underlying reasons for pursuing your goals can reinvigorate your enthusiasm and dedication. Remind yourself of the benefits that achieving these goals will bring to your life, and allow this vision to drive you forward through challenging periods.

Incorporating these strategies into your approach prepares you for potential setbacks and empowers you to move forward confidently, knowing you have a plan to handle the ups and downs effectively. By anticipating challenges, setting preventive measures, building flexibility, and maintaining motivation, you create a robust framework that supports sustained effort and success in managing long-term commitments with ADHD.

As this chapter closes, we reflect on the importance of foresight and preparation in managing long-term projects with ADHD. The strategies discussed serve as a guide to anticipate challenges and equip yourself with tools to navigate them effectively. Looking ahead, these foundational skills pave the way for tackling more complex tasks and achieving greater aspirations, which we will explore in the forthcoming chapters. With each step, you are not just planning and anticipating; you are setting the stage for a life where ADHD does not dictate your limits but enhances your journey toward personal and professional fulfillment.

7

LIFESTYLE ADJUSTMENTS FOR OPTIMAL TIME MANAGEMENT

Imagine navigating through a dense forest, where each tree represents a unique challenge or distraction. Now, envision having a clear path marked out, one that guides you through the thickest underbrush directly to your desired destination. This is the power of effective lifestyle adjustments for your time 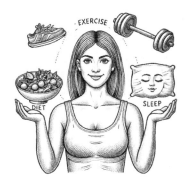 management, especially when you're dealing with ADHD. It's about creating an internal and external environment that enhances your ability to focus, make decisions, and move forward confidently.

In this chapter, we focus on the foundational trio of diet, exercise, and sleep—elements that are crucial not just for managing ADHD but for transforming how you interact with time and tasks every day. By making these adjustments, you're taking control of your life and your ADHD, and that's a powerful thing.

DIET, EXERCISE, AND SLEEP: THE TRIFECTA FOR BETTER FOCUS

Nutritional Choices and Brain Function

The food you eat plays a pivotal role in how well you can focus and manage your time. Think of your brain as an orchestra conductor, directing numerous instruments that create the symphony of your daily actions, thoughts, and decisions. Just like a conductor needs a clear podium from which to lead, your brain needs the right kind of fuel to function optimally. For those with ADHD, certain foods can help reduce hyperactivity and enhance focus.

Protein-rich foods, for example, are essential. They provide the amino acids your body uses to produce neurotransmitters, such as dopamine and norepinephrine, which are crucial for attention and thinking. Starting your day with a protein-packed breakfast can help maintain stable blood sugar levels, which is vital for preventing mid-morning crashes that affect your focus. Foods rich in omega-3 fatty acids, like salmon, walnuts, and flaxseeds, are also beneficial. Omega-3s are vital components of brain cell membranes and are known for their role in enhancing brain function, particularly regarding memory and mood stabilization.

Incorporating these nutritional elements into your diet involves not only adding specific foods but also maintaining consistency and balance. Planning your meals can prevent impulsive eating, often leading to less-than-ideal choices for brain health. Consider using a meal-planning app or tool to help you organize your weekly meals, ensuring that you have the right ingredients to create meals that support your cognitive function and manage your ADHD.

Exercise as a Tool for Focus

Regular physical activity is another cornerstone of effective time management for those with ADHD. Exercise isn't just about physical health; it's a potent stimulant for the brain, releasing crucial chemicals for attention, memory, and mood. Engaging in regular exercise can help alleviate common symptoms of ADHD, such as inattention, hyperactivity, and impulsivity. Aerobic activities, like jogging, swimming, or cycling, are particularly effective as they increase heart rate and blood flow to the brain, enhancing neural connectivity and efficacy.

Martial arts and yoga can also be highly beneficial, especially for their focus on discipline, structure, and mindfulness—qualities that can directly translate into better time management skills. These activities require mental engagement and body awareness to help train your brain to focus more effectively, even outside physical exercise sessions.

Incorporating exercise into your daily routine can be a manageable task. It can be as simple as a morning walk or cycling after work. The key is to find an activity you enjoy, making it more likely that you will stick to it. Remember, consistency is crucial; regular physical activity accumulates benefits over time, not just in physical health but also in your cognitive and time management capabilities.

The Role of Sleep in Managing ADHD

Sleep is perhaps the most underrated tool in managing ADHD and enhancing time management. Lack of quality sleep can worsen symptoms of ADHD, such as inattention, impulsivity, and distractibility. Ensuring you get enough restful sleep is crucial for your brain to function optimally. During sleep, your brain processes the day's learning and experiences, forms memories, and clears out toxins. This vital process is essential for cognitive functions that affect time management, such as decision-making, problem-solving, and emotional regulation.

Creating a bedtime routine that promotes restful sleep is vital. This might include winding down activities an hour before bed, such as reading or listening to calming music and avoiding stimulating activities like watching TV or scrolling through social media. Keeping your bedroom cool, dark, and quiet can also enhance sleep quality. If sleep remains elusive, consider consulting a healthcare provider to explore possible underlying causes and solutions. Sometimes, ADHD medications or co-existing conditions like anxiety can interfere with sleep, and addressing these issues can significantly improve sleep quality and, by extension, your time management.

Integrating Healthy Habits

Incorporating nutritional choices, regular physical activity, and quality sleep into your daily life requires intention and planning. But the benefits to your time management and overall well-being are immense. Start small by changing one meal daily to include more brain-boosting foods or introducing a 10-minute walk into your routine. Gradually build on these changes as they become habitual. Remember, the goal is to create a lifestyle that supports your ability to focus, manage time, and reduce the symptoms of ADHD. By making thoughtful adjustments to your diet, exercise, and sleep habits, you're not only improving your time management but also setting the foundation for a healthier, more focused version of yourself. These changes are about more than just small improvements—they're about creating a better, more balanced you.

Visual Element: Infographic on Building a Healthy ADHD-Friendly Routine

To help you visualize and implement these lifestyle changes, consider creating an infographic that outlines the steps to building a healthy, ADHD-friendly routine. It provides a visual summary of the key points discussed, offering a quick reference to help you remember and apply these strategies in your daily life. The infographic includes tips on integrating brain-healthy foods into your diet, ideas for incorporating exercise into your schedule, and suggestions for establishing a restful bedtime routine. Use this tool as a daily reminder of the small changes you can make that lead to significant improvements in managing your time and enhancing your focus.

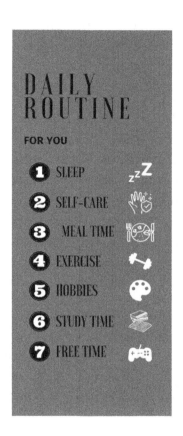

THE IMPACT OF PHYSICAL ORGANIZATION ON TIME MANAGEMENT

Physical clutter is a mere annoyance and a significant hurdle, adding complexity to your cognitive processes. It's like trying to navigate through a crowded room filled with obstacles; every additional item in your way demands attention, saps energy, and complicates your path forward. This phenomenon, known as cognitive overload, can be particularly debilitating for individuals with ADHD, as it amplifies common symptoms such as distractibility, forgetfulness, and overwhelm. When your environment is cluttered, your brain, already taxed with the effort to focus and organize thoughts, has to work even harder to filter through unnecessary stimuli, leading to decreased productivity and heightened stress.

To combat these effects, creating organized physical spaces is crucial. Start with a clear assessment of your most-used spaces—your desk, kitchen, or digital workspace. Identify what items are essential and what are merely occupying valuable space. Begin decluttering by removing items you haven't used in the last 6 months. This can be challenging, as the decision-making process might trigger anxiety or indecision, familiar companions of ADHD. To ease this, use a systematic approach: sort items into categories, such as "keep," "discard," and "donate," and tackle one category at a time to avoid feeling overwhelmed.

Once you've streamlined your possessions, consider implementing organizational systems catering to ADHD needs. These systems should be simple and visually straightforward, minimizing the need for complex decision-making. Use clear, labeled containers for physical items to reduce visual clutter and make it easy to find what you need. For paperwork and digital files, adopt a straightforward filing system—alphabetical, chronological, or by project—whichever makes the most sense for your thoughts and work. Regularly scheduled "maintenance" sessions can help keep this system in order, preventing clutter from accumulating again. For instance, dedicating 10 minutes at the end of each day to tidy your workspace can make a significant difference in managing clutter and maintaining organization.

Ergonomically friendly environments are another critical aspect of optimizing your space for better focus and productivity. The physical arrangement of your workspace can significantly impact your ability to concentrate and work effectively. An ergonomically designed workspace reduces physical strain and supports sustained attention, which is particularly beneficial when you have ADHD. Ensure that your chair supports your back comfortably, your desk is at an appropriate height, and your computer monitor is positioned to reduce eye strain. Incorporate elements that enhance focus, such as natural lighting or noise-canceling headphones.

Maintaining an organized environment requires consistent effort, especially when ADHD is part of the equation. Strategies for regular maintenance of physical organization include setting reminders to clean and organize at specific intervals or incorporating cleaning into your daily routines as a habitual practice. Visual cues can also be beneficial; for example, a small sign that says "5-minute tidy-up" placed in a prominent spot can remind you to take brief, regular breaks to maintain order in your workspace. Remember, the goal of these practices isn't just to keep your space tidy but to create an environment that significantly enhances your ability to manage time and tasks effectively.

By taking control of your physical surroundings, you're organizing your space and setting the stage for a clearer mind and a more focused approach to every task you undertake. This doesn't mean your space has to be stark or devoid of personality; instead, it's about creating an environment that resonates with your style while promoting efficiency and calm. Whether it's through decluttering, adopting ergonomic practices, or setting up simple, sustainable organizational systems, your changes can profoundly impact reducing cognitive overload and enhancing your overall productivity and well-being.

MINIMALISM AND ADHD: REDUCING CLUTTER TO ENHANCE FOCUS

Embracing minimalism might initially seem like just another trend, but for individuals with ADHD, it represents a profound shift toward clarity and simplicity. The essence of minimalism lies in eliminating the unnecessary, allowing you to focus on what truly matters. This philosophy can be particularly impactful if your attention is often scattered or overwhelmed by the abundance of physical and digital clutter. By reducing the stimuli in your environment, minimalism helps limit distractions and simplifies decision-making processes, making daily life more manageable and less stressful.

Minimalism is more than just having fewer things—it's about intentional living, encouraging you to question what items and activities add value to your life. For someone with ADHD, this can mean the difference between feeling overwhelmed by too many choices and feeling empowered by selecting just what is truly essential. Minimalism fosters a sense of physical and mental space, which can be incredibly freeing. It's about creating room for your mind to breathe and focus, enhancing your ability to concentrate on tasks without the constant tug of clutter pulling your attention away.

Applying minimalism in your life starts with the physical spaces you inhabit. Begin by decluttering your living and working areas. This doesn't mean you need to strip everything back to bare walls and floors, but rather, carefully choose what deserves a place in your space. Each item in your environment should serve a purpose or bring joy; everything else is potentially a distraction. For instance, focusing on work can be challenging if your desk is cluttered with papers, gadgets, and miscellaneous items. By clearing out unnecessary items and organizing what remains into a simple, efficient system, you create a workspace that supports productivity rather than hinders it.

Expanding minimalism into the digital realm can also dramatically improve your focus and time management. Digital clutter, from unused apps on your phone to a desktop littered with icons, can be just as distracting as physical clutter. Start by decluttering your digital devices. Uninstall apps you no longer use, organize files into clearly labeled folders, and keep your desktop icons to a minimum. Reducing the number of notifications you receive daily can also decrease digital noise, allowing you to concentrate better. Managing your social media consumption by setting specific times for checking platforms or using apps that limit your usage can free up considerable mental space and reduce the urge to switch tasks constantly.

Minimalism also extends to how you manage your time. By applying minimalist principles to your scheduling, you can avoid overcommitting and reduce feeling overwhelmed. Prioritize your tasks based on the most important or urgent, and be realistic about what you can achieve daily. This might mean saying "no" to requests that do not align with your priorities or delegating tasks when possible. Think of it as making space in your schedule for activities that add value to your life, whether work, hobbies, or rest. Creating a minimalist schedule isn't about doing less for the sake of less; it's about doing enough of what matters most to you, leading to greater satisfaction and better time management.

Let's consider two individuals who have embraced minimalism and seen significant improvements in their lives. First, meet Alex, a writer with ADHD who always felt overwhelmed by his chaotic home office. After adopting a minimalist approach, Alex removed all non-essential items from his workspace, organized his remaining tools into easily accessible places, and digitized his paperwork to reduce physical clutter. This transformation allowed him to focus intensely when writing, increasing productivity and significantly reducing his daily stress.

Then there's Emma, a software developer who struggled with digital distractions. By decluttering her computer desktop, uninstalling unnecessary apps, and using a website blocker during work hours, Emma minimized digital distractions significantly. She also adopted a minimalist approach to her daily tasks, focusing only on the essential tasks that would advance her projects. This boosted her productivity and allowed her more time to enjoy leisure activities, which improved her overall wellbeing.

These examples illustrate the tangible benefits of applying minimalism across various aspects of life. Whether clearing your physical or digital workspace or simplifying your daily schedule, minimalism offers a powerful strategy for enhancing focus and efficiency, particularly for individuals with ADHD.

ESTABLISHING ROUTINES THAT STICK: TIPS AND TRICKS

Why do routines resonate so profoundly with managing ADHD? It boils down to the brain's love for patterns and predictability, which counteracts the characteristic unpredictability of ADHD. Establishing a routine is akin to setting tracks for a train—the locomotive will follow the predetermined path, reducing the need for constant steering and adjustments. For you, routines can automate decision-making processes, significantly reducing the cognitive load of planning and initiating tasks. This automation is crucial because it conserves your mental energy, allowing you to focus more on execution rather than getting bogged down by the details of starting each task anew daily.

Creating effective routines, however, is not about rigidly structuring every moment of your day but rather about finding a balance that accommodates the variable nature of ADHD. The key is to identify core activities that benefit most from routinization—those that are essential but perhaps mundane or those that you tend to procrastinate on. Begin by mapping out a typical day and pinpointing where you feel most overwhelmed or tend to drift off track. These are your targets for routinization. For instance, if mornings are chaotic, a structured start involving simple tasks like making your bed, having a nutritious breakfast, and planning your day can set a positive tone for hours ahead.

Implementing these routines requires support, particularly in tools and apps that remind you of what comes next until the sequence becomes a natural part of your day. Apps like Habitica or Todoist can be programmed to nudge you at specific times, reinforcing your new habits. They can also help track your progress, giving you a visual representation of your consistency, which can be incredibly motivating. Remember, using these tools is not to create additional stress but to serve as gentle reminders that help you stay aligned with your intentions.

Adjusting your routines is just as important as setting them up. Life is dynamic—your needs and circumstances can change, and your routines should evolve. Regular reviews of your routines every few months can be beneficial. Assess what's working and what isn't, and don't hesitate to tweak your routines to better suit your current lifestyle or goals. This might mean shifting your exercise routine from evening to morning if it energizes your day or adjusting your work routine to accommodate a new project or job.

Understanding that routines are fluid, not static, will help you maintain them in the long run. They are meant to support your life, not constrain it. By finding the right balance, integrating supportive tools, and being willing to make adjustments, you can transform your daily routines from a source of stress to a foundation of stability and focus in managing your ADHD. This proactive approach enhances your daily productivity and improves your overall quality of life, making navigating the challenges easier and capitalizing on the strengths of living with ADHD.

As we wrap up this segment on establishing effective routines, remember that the essence of this guidance is to simplify your life, not complicate it. These routines reduce the everyday chaos that can cloud your mind and hinder your productivity. They are your stepping stones to a more organized, focused, and fulfilling life. Embrace these strategies with an open mind and adapt them as you go along. What works for others might not work for you, and that's perfectly okay. The goal is to find what best helps you thrive.

In the next chapter, we'll explore how leveraging your interpersonal skills can significantly enhance your time management strategies, turning everyday interactions into opportunities for growth and efficiency.

8

COMMUNICATING AND COLLABORATING WITH OTHERS

Imagine standing on a stage, spotlight shining down, with an audience of peers, family, and colleagues before you. They're here to understand your unique approach to managing time, influenced by your experience with ADHD. This chapter is about equipping you with the skills to confidently explain 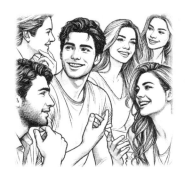 your time management needs, transforming potential misunderstandings into opportunities for support and collaboration. Understanding and articulating your needs effectively is crucial for fostering better relationships and creating a supportive network that recognizes and adapts to your unique requirements, ultimately enhancing your productivity and well-being. It involves making sure your voice is heard and your needs are respected.

EXPLAINING YOUR TIME MANAGEMENT NEEDS TO OTHERS

Importance of Open Communication

In personal and professional realms, transparent and open communication is the cornerstone of understanding and cooperation. For adults with ADHD, where time management can be a daily challenge, explaining your specific needs to those around you is crucial. This openness not only helps set realistic expectations, inviting others to offer the proper support or adjustments, but it also empowers you. By articulating your needs, you're providing a manual on the best ways to collaborate with you effectively, ensuring that both your needs and the needs of others are met harmoniously. This empowerment is crucial to effectively communicate your time management needs.

Tips for Articulating Needs

Communicating your time management challenges effectively requires clarity and confidence. Start by clearly defining your own needs and challenges. Understand what aspects of time management you struggle with, whether maintaining focus, estimating how long tasks will take, or handling multitasking. Once you have a clear grasp, articulate these challenges to others without downplaying or exaggerating—just the plain realities. Use simple, direct language and, if possible, relate your needs to your mutual goals. For instance, you might explain to a colleague, "I use tools like digital reminders and task lists to keep track of deadlines. Aligning our project timelines with these tools helps me ensure I'm contributing effectively."

Role-Playing to Build Confidence

Consider engaging in role-playing exercises to build confidence in discussing your ADHD-related time management needs. You can practice with a friend or family member or even in front of a mirror. Set up a scenario, such as explaining your time management strategies during a team meeting or discussing your needs with a new project partner. Role-playing can help refine your delivery, making you more comfortable when you need to have these real-life conversations. It also prepares you to respond to various reactions, from supportive to skeptical, ensuring that you remain composed and persuasive no matter the response.

Creating Informative Materials

Sometimes, words need reinforcement through tangible materials that others can refer to. Creating concise, informative materials such as a one-pager or a brief presentation can be extremely helpful, especially in professional settings. These materials should outline key points about ADHD and its impact on time management, your specific strategies, and how others can support them. For instance, a one-pager for your manager could include a brief description of ADHD, an overview of your preferred tools (like specific apps or methods), and a list of potential adjustments in work processes that could help you perform better, such as flexible deadlines or a quiet workspace.

Interactive Element: Communication Practice Worksheet

To further aid in your communication efforts, consider using a structured worksheet where you can script and refine what you want to say. This worksheet should include sections for:

- **Your Time Management Challenges:** Briefly describe your main challenges.
- **Your Strategies:** List the tools and techniques you use to manage your time.
- **Needs From Others:** Specify what adjustments or support you need from others.
- **Potential Questions/Reactions:** Prepare responses for possible questions or reactions you might encounter.

This exercise helps you organize your thoughts and ensure you cover all necessary points during your discussions, making your communication as effective as possible. By approaching conversations about your ADHD and time management needs with clarity and preparedness, you foster an environment of understanding and support, enhancing your personal interactions and professional collaborations.

STRATEGIES FOR EFFECTIVE TEAMWORK AND DELEGATION

When you work within a team, understanding how to leverage each member's strengths, including your own, can transform collective output and streamline project completion. This is especially pivotal when managing ADHD, where diverse talents can complement your unique approach to handling tasks. Start by conducting an open and honest assessment of each team member's skills and preferences. This doesn't just help in assigning roles more effectively but fosters an environment where everyone's capabilities are fully utilized, boosting overall team morale and efficiency. For instance, if a team member excels at data analysis but struggles with public speaking, assigning them to handle backend research rather than leading client presentations plays to their strengths and maintains the team's productivity.

Delegation is a critical skill in any team setting but can be particularly challenging when you have ADHD. It involves not only deciding which tasks to delegate but also to whom. For those with ADHD, the key is to delegate tasks that might be more routine or require attention to detail that could be taxing due to your ADHD symptoms. Identify tasks that align with your team member's strengths and interests. This ensures the task is likely to be completed well and builds trust and respect within the team. When delegating, be clear about the task and your expectations for completion. This clarity helps prevent misunderstandings and ensures the work is done correctly and efficiently.

In today's digital age, leveraging technology effectively can significantly enhance team collaboration, especially for individuals with ADHD who benefit from structured and clear communication. Tools like Slack for instant messaging, Trello for task management, and Zoom for virtual meetings can keep everyone on the same page. These tools are not just handy; they are reassuring because they allow you to create a shared workspace where tasks, updates, and deadlines are visible to all team members, reducing the cognitive load on any single person and ensuring that everyone knows what needs to be done, when, and by whom. Additionally, many of these tools offer features like reminders and notifications that can be invaluable for managing ADHD symptoms that might otherwise lead to forgetfulness or oversight. This emphasis on the supportive role of technology can make the audience feel reassured and confident in their ability to manage their time effectively.

Maintaining accountability within a team is crucial, mainly when tasks are delegated. One effective method is to set up regular check-ins or updates. This could be as simple as a brief daily stand-up meeting where team members report on their progress and highlight any challenges they face. These meetings help align the team and allow you to offer support or resources that might be needed to keep the project moving forward. Additionally, a shared digital calendar or project management tool where tasks and deadlines are clearly noted and progress is tracked visibly can help ensure everyone is accountable for their parts. This visibility motivates team members and allows for early identification of potential delays or issues, which can be addressed before they become problematic.

Incorporating these strategies into your team interactions can significantly affect how effectively you work together and achieve your goals. By understanding and leveraging individual strengths, using the right tools to facilitate communication and coordination, and keeping everyone accountable, you can create a dynamic team environment that accommodates your ADHD and enhances the productivity and satisfaction of the entire team. As you continue to apply these strategies, you likely find that not only are your projects completed more efficiently, but the stress and chaos often associated with group work are significantly reduced, leaving more room for creativity and innovation.

HANDLING CRITICISM AND MISUNDERSTANDINGS ABOUT YOUR TIME MANAGEMENT

Criticism, especially when it touches on aspects of our lives that we struggle with, like time management in the context of ADHD, can feel particularly personal and disheartening. The impact of criticism lies not only in the words spoken but also in the emotions and doubts they provoke within us. However, transforming how we receive and respond to such feedback can turn these challenging moments into opportunities for growth, self-awareness, and improved understanding of others. When criticism comes your way, particularly about time management, the first step is to process it constructively. View it through a more analytical lens instead of internalizing it as a personal failure. Ask yourself whether the feedback is rooted in observable facts and consider the intent behind it. Sometimes, criticism may come across as a misguided attempt to help. It's crucial to discern the difference between feedback that is meant to be constructive and comments that are purely critical without any basis for improvement.

To effectively handle such feedback, start by taking a moment to breathe and center yourself, preventing an immediate, possibly emotional reaction. This pause allows you to approach the situation more calmly and thoughtfully. Next, seek to understand the perspective of the person providing the feedback. Ask clarifying questions if necessary. This helps you grasp the full context of the feedback and shows the other person that you are open to dialogue, which can diffuse potential conflict and lead to more productive exchanges. Once you fully understand the feedback, evaluate its validity and relevance to your goals and strategies. If the feedback is useful, consider how to incorporate it into your time management practices. If it's not, be prepared to explain why, ideally in a way that helps the critic see your point of view.

Misconceptions about ADHD can often underlie criticisms of your time management, making it crucial to address and clarify them whenever they arise. Many people still equate ADHD with simple distractibility or disorganization, not understanding the complex ways it affects cognition and behavior, including time perception and management. When faced with criticism from such misconceptions, take the opportunity to educate the other person about ADHD. Explain, for instance, how time blindness might affect your ability to adhere strictly to schedules or how hyperfocus might lead you to lose track of time. Providing specific examples can help make these concepts more concrete for the listener, fostering greater empathy and understanding.

Building emotional resilience is essential in handling criticism and in all areas of life where ADHD plays a role. This resilience can buffer against the stress and emotional turbulence that might otherwise exacerbate ADHD symptoms, leading to a vicious cycle of stress and decreased productivity. Strengthening your emotional resilience involves regular self-care practices, such as mindfulness meditation, which has been shown to reduce emotional reactivity. It also involves building a solid support network of friends, family, or even a professional therapist who understands and supports your ADHD management efforts. These resources provide emotional comfort, practical advice, and perspectives that must be added to your considerations.

Finally, always aim for constructive dialogue, especially when navigating criticisms or misunderstandings. This means actively listening, being open to other perspectives, and responding thoughtfully. Approach each conversation with the goal of mutual understanding rather than winning an argument. Effective communication strategies, such as using "I" statements to express your feelings rather than accusatory "you" statements, can help keep discussions positive and productive.

Remember, every conversation is an opportunity to improve understanding, strengthen relationships, and refine your approaches to managing your time and ADHD. By embracing these principles, you empower yourself and those around you, creating a more supportive and understanding environment for managing your ADHD effectively.

BUILDING EMPATHY: HELPING OTHERS UNDERSTAND
ADHD

In bridging the gap between personal experiences with ADHD and
the perceptions held by others, education stands as a pivotal tool.
By illuminating the multifaceted nature of ADHD, we can transform misunderstanding into empathy, fostering environments
where diversity in cognitive styles is accepted and appreciated.

Educating others about ADHD involves more than sharing facts;
it's about reshaping narratives and highlighting the nuanced experiences of those living with the condition. Start by introducing
foundational knowledge about ADHD in a way that resonates
personally. Workshops, informal discussions, and even digital
content such as webinars can effectively spread awareness. When
discussing ADHD, emphasize the spectrum of symptoms and the
variability of experiences—it's not the same for everyone.
Tailoring this information to your audience—whether they are
colleagues, family members, or educators—ensures that the
message is heard and understood. For instance, when talking to
employers, focus on how ADHD traits can be channeled into
unique strengths in the workplace, such as creativity and problem-
solving.

Sharing personal stories is another powerful method to foster
empathy and break down the stigmas associated with ADHD.
Stories humanize the challenges and triumphs of living with
ADHD, making the abstract symptoms more tangible. Encourage
individuals with ADHD to share their journeys at support groups,
through social media, or in community forums. These narratives
can profoundly impact listeners, altering perceptions and encouraging a more compassionate viewpoint. For example, sharing how
you turned a hyperfocus trait into a professional asset during a

team meeting can enlighten colleagues about the positive aspects of ADHD, challenging preconceived notions.

Advocating for environments that support neurodiversity involves actively creating inclusive spaces in professional and social settings. This advocacy can take many forms, from initiating policy changes in the workplace that accommodate neurodiverse employees to supporting local businesses that implement ADHD-friendly practices. Within the workplace, this might look like proposing modifications to the physical and cultural environment that help reduce sensory overload—a common challenge for those with ADHD. Simple changes, such as providing noise-canceling headphones or creating quiet work zones, can significantly affect productivity and well-being.

Leveraging existing networks that support ADHD and neurodiversity plays a crucial role in building broader empathy and understanding. Many communities and online platforms offer resources, advice, and support for individuals with ADHD and their allies. By engaging with these networks, you can amplify their messages and advocate for greater awareness and support across various settings. Participate in forums, attend conferences, or volunteer with organizations dedicated to neurodiversity to stay informed and connected. These activities strengthen your knowledge and support network and position you to effectively educate others about the realities of living with ADHD.

Through these efforts, we educate, share, and build bridges of understanding that can transform everyday interactions and societal perceptions of ADHD. Each conversation, story, and informed gesture contributes to a more empathetic and inclusive world where the diverse tapestries of human cognition are fully valued. As we move forward, let's carry the insights from these discussions into our daily lives, continuing to advocate for understanding and support in every environment we inhabit.

In wrapping up this chapter, we've navigated the delicate yet crucial process of building empathy and understanding around ADHD. From educational efforts that demystify the condition to personal stories that connect on a human level, each step is a stride toward a more inclusive society. As we continue into the next chapter, we carry forward the principles of empathy and understanding, exploring how they can be translated into practical strategies for managing daily tasks and long-term goals.

9

TAILORING TRADITIONAL TIME MANAGEMENT TO FIT ADHD

Imagine standing in a library filled with every book on time management ever written, yet none of them seem to speak your language. This is often how traditional time management strategies can feel to someone with ADHD. They offer solid advice, sure, but they don't always account for the whirlwind of distractions, the sudden dips in 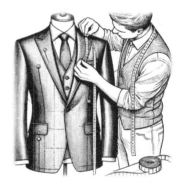 motivation, or the unique way your mind processes time.

This chapter is about reshaping these traditional tools so they work for you, not against you. It's about making the principles of time management dance to the rhythm of your ADHD, creating a symphony where there once was discord. By customizing these tools, you're taking control and showing the world what you're capable of.

CUSTOMIZING THE BULLET JOURNAL APPROACH FOR ADHD

Introduction to the Bullet Journal

The Bullet Journal, created by Ryder Carroll, a digital product designer, is a flexible organization system that combines tasks, notes, reflections, and calendar events into a straightforward notebook. It's hailed for its simplicity and efficiency, appealing especially to those who crave structure but still want the freedom to customize their organizational tools. At its core, the Bullet Journal uses rapid logging—symbols, shorthand notations, and short sentences to capture information quickly. For many, it's more than just a productivity tool; it's a mindfulness practice disguised as a notebook.

ADHD-Specific Customizations

However, for those with ADHD, the traditional Bullet Journal layout might need some tweaking to truly fit your needs. Color coding, for instance, can be a game-changer. Assigning different colors to various tasks (e.g., blue for work, green for personal, yellow for appointments) makes your journal more visually appealing. It helps process and segregate information quickly—a frequent need for ADHD minds that might feel overwhelmed by too much data.

Simplified symbols or notations can further reduce the cognitive load. Instead of complex icons that might be difficult to remember, opt for simple bullets, dashes, or checks. This modification ensures that you spend less time recalling what each symbol means and doing the tasks more.

Structured templates are another crucial customization. While the Bullet Journal champions flexibility, having templates for daily, weekly, or monthly pages can provide the scaffolding necessary to guide your ADHD brain. Templates can help ensure consistency and completeness, reducing the anxiety of where to start or what to write.

Incorporating Flexibility

Flexibility in a Bullet Journal is vital for adapting to the often unpredictable productivity levels associated with ADHD. This means setting up your journal to handle changes without much hassle. For example, instead of pre-dating each page, you leave the dates blank and fill them in as you go, allowing you to skip days without the guilt of leaving blank pages. Similarly, using a binder-style notebook where pages can be easily added or removed can accommodate the ebb and flow of your energy and focus.

Examples and Case Studies

Consider the story of Alex, a graphic designer with ADHD, who struggled with traditional planners that felt rigid and uninspiring. He decided to create his own Bullet Journal, customizing it to fit his unique needs. Alex used color-coded tasks and flexible layouts, choosing the colors and designs that resonated with him. This personalized approach allowed him to track project deadlines and personal appointments in a way that felt intuitive and engaging. The visual variety helped him quickly locate specific tasks, and the ability to rearrange pages meant he could manage his fluctuating productivity without feeling restricted by a pre-set format.

Similarly, consider Emily, a freelance writer who struggled to find a planning system that worked for her diverse and demanding projects. She experimented with various tools, starting with a traditional planner, but found it too rigid for her needs. She then tried digital apps, which offered flexibility but lacked the tactile satisfaction she craved.

Finally, Emily discovered the Bullet Journal and decided to customize it to suit her workflow. She began by breaking down her large writing projects into bite-sized tasks, experimenting with different ways to track her progress. Eventually, she settled on color-coding each phase—research, drafting, editing, and submitting—using her favorite shades to make the process more engaging. This system gave her a clear visual of where she stood with each project, turning overwhelming tasks into manageable steps.

Emily also adapted her daily template, incorporating time blocks for deep focus work, which she discovered through trial and error. This adjustment aligned perfectly with her natural workflow, allowing her to better manage her time and meet deadlines without feeling overwhelmed. Over time, she augmented her Bullet Journal with sticky notes for quick reminders and a digital calendar for appointment alerts, creating a hybrid system that balanced her need for both structure and creativity.

These adaptations are not just about making the Bullet Journal prettier or more organized; they are about aligning a popular productivity system with the specific needs of the ADHD brain. By customizing this method, Alex, Sarah, and many others have found a way to make time management a personalized, responsive tool that genuinely supports their daily lives and boosts their productivity.

TIME MANAGEMENT MYTHS VS. REALITY FOR ADHD

In the vast ocean of time management advice, certain myths persist that may not necessarily hold up under the unique pressures and characteristics of ADHD. It's crucial to differentiate between general advice and what actually applies to you, mainly when myths like the effectiveness of multitasking or adhering to a rigid schedule are often perpetuated as universal truths. The reality is, for many with ADHD, these common time management strategies can do more harm than good, leading to increased stress and decreased productivity. By debunking these myths, you can feel reassured that you're not alone in your struggles and enlightened about the strategies that truly work for you.

Debunking Common Myths

Let's tackle the myth of multitasking first. It's popular that doing multiple tasks at once can increase efficiency. However, for someone with ADHD, multitasking can lead to divided attention, half-completed tasks, and increased mental clutter. Research suggests that what is often thought of as multitasking is task-switching, and each switch can cause a decline in performance. For those with ADHD, whose executive functions are already taxed, the additional cognitive load can lead to errors and frustration. Instead, focusing on one task at a time—a strategy known as "single-tasking"—can increase efficiency and reduce the overwhelm that often accompanies multitasking.

Another pervasive myth is the need for a rigid daily schedule. While structure is beneficial, too rigid an approach can be impractical for someone with ADHD, whose day-to-day functionality can vary significantly. Flexibility is key. It's about finding a balance that allows for the natural ebb and flow of energy and focus that characterizes ADHD. Structured flexibility—having a plan but allowing for adjustments based on your mental and physical state —is often more effective. This approach reduces the guilt and stress associated with failing to stick to a strict schedule, which can be a significant emotional drain for those with ADHD.

ADHD Reality Check

Addressing what time management realistically looks like for someone with ADHD is crucial for setting practical and achievable goals. It often involves a series of trial and error, discovering what methods resonate with your experience of ADHD. Common challenges include inconsistent productivity levels, where one day might be filled with high energy and focus, followed by a period where completing even minor tasks feels daunting. Recognizing and planning for these fluctuations can lead to a more realistic approach to time management. Remember, it's a journey of continuous improvement, and each step forward brings you closer to a more efficient and manageable way of living with ADHD.

Moreover, external distractions and internal restlessness can significantly hinder effective time management. Strategies we've already discussed, such as noise-canceling headphones, creating a minimally distracting workspace, or using apps that limit internet access, can be beneficial. These tools help create an environment that supports focus and minimizes the impact of ADHD symptoms on productivity.

Educating Others

When it comes to educating those around you—be it peers, family, or employers—about managing time with ADHD, clarity and honesty are vital. Explaining the realities of ADHD can help set realistic expectations and foster a supportive environment. It's helpful to describe how ADHD affects your time management, perhaps explaining the need for breaks to maintain focus or why a flexible schedule is necessary. Offering solutions or adjustments that can help improve productivity, such as periodic check-ins instead of long meetings, can also be beneficial.

Sharing resources, such as articles, books, or videos about ADHD and time management, can help others understand your needs and the strategies that assist you. This educates and empowers those around you to provide the proper support, which can make a significant difference in personal and professional realms.

Balancing Expectations and Abilities

Finally, balancing your expectations with your abilities is crucial for effective time management. This means setting goals that are challenging yet achievable, considering ADHD's variable nature. Celebrating small victories along the way is essential, as this can boost confidence and motivation. For instance, if completing a project on time is challenging, breaking it down into smaller, more manageable tasks and setting mini-deadlines provide a sense of accomplishment as each segment is completed.

Moreover, be honest with yourself about what is feasible. Overcommitting can lead to stress and a sense of failure. Learn to gauge what you can realistically handle, and don't hesitate to adjust your commitments as needed. This self-awareness is critical to managing time effectively and maintaining mental health and well-being.

In essence, managing time with ADHD requires a nuanced under-standing of both the condition and the individual ways it manifests in your life. By debunking myths, adjusting expectations, and educating those around you, you can create a framework for time management that respects your unique needs and leverages your strengths.

INTEGRATING ADHD NEEDS INTO EXISTING TIME MANAGEMENT SYSTEMS

Stepping into the realm of traditional time management systems often feels like trying to fit a square peg into a round hole, especially when you're dealing with ADHD. Systems like Getting Things Done (GTD) by David Allen or the Eisenhower Box offer robust frameworks to streamline efficiency and productivity. However, without the proper modifications, these systems can sometimes overlook the unique challenges that come with ADHD, such as fluctuating energy levels, difficulty with sustained attention, and the need for frequent stimulation.

Assessment of Popular Systems

Let's start by assessing how these popular systems align with ADHD needs. GTD, for instance, is a method that emphasizes capturing all your tasks in a trusted system outside your brain and then breaking them down into actionable steps organized by context. While this method promotes externalizing your tasks—which can be particularly beneficial if you struggle with working memory—the capture phase can be overwhelming. Without modifications, the sheer volume of capturing every "unfinished task" can lead to cognitive overload.

On the other hand, the Eisenhower Box, which divides tasks into categories based on urgency and importance, offers a clear visual framework for prioritization. Yet, for someone with ADHD, the challenge often lies in accurately assessing the urgency and importance of each task due to impairments in executive function. This can lead to misplacing tasks in inappropriate quadrants, thereby skewing priorities.

Custom Integration Techniques

To better tailor these systems to ADHD, consider integrating visual aids and simplifying processes. Using color-coded cards or digital tags for the Eisenhower Box can help visually distinguish between quadrants. This makes it easier to see where your tasks lie at a glance and taps into the ADHD brain's preference for color and visuals, which can enhance engagement and memory.

In GTD, simplifying the capture phase can prevent feelings of overwhelm. Instead of trying to record every task and thought immediately, you might set specific times throughout the day for batch processing. During these times, use a digital recorder or a simple note-taking app to quickly dump your thoughts, which you can later sort and process. This method reduces the pressure to capture everything perfectly on the first go, a common source of anxiety for many with ADHD.

Using Technology to Enhance Systems

Technology can be a powerful ally in making these traditional systems work for you. Numerous apps and tools are designed to complement methodologies like GTD and the Eisenhower Box. For instance, apps like Todoist or Asana can be customized to mirror the GTD framework but with features that cater to ADHD, such as customizable notifications, recurring reminders, and visual project trackers. These features can help maintain momentum and ensure nothing falls through the cracks.

Furthermore, integrating these apps with other tech tools that you use daily, like calendar apps or digital notebooks, can create a seamless ecosystem where all your information is interconnected. This saves time and reduces the mental effort required to switch between different tools, a common barrier to sustaining focus.

Personalization Tips

The key to successfully integrating these systems into your life lies in personalization. Start by identifying which elements resonate with you and which ones trigger your ADHD symptoms. Experiment with different adaptations and observe what helps reduce friction and increase flow in your work. Remember, the goal is not to rigidly adhere to these systems but to use them as scaffolds, adapting their structures to meet your unique needs.

A hybrid approach works best: Use the GTD method for work-related tasks but switch to the Eisenhower Box for personal projects. You'll also discover that some aspects of these systems can be combined or modified to create a customized framework that feels right for you.

Ultimately, integrating your ADHD needs into existing time management systems is not about conforming to an idealized productivity standard. It's about crafting a personal productivity system that acknowledges and accommodates your unique brain wiring, allowing you to manage your time and tasks naturally and sustainably. By taking the time to understand and modify these systems, you empower yourself to navigate your days with confidence and clarity, turning time management from a daunting chore into an empowering tool that supports your journey.

CONTINUOUS IMPROVEMENT: EVOLVING YOUR STRATEGIES AS NEEDS CHANGE

In the dynamic landscape of managing ADHD, the only constant is change. As you navigate through various phases of life, your needs, challenges, and the effectiveness of your strategies will inevitably shift. Embracing a mindset of continuous improvement in managing your time is beneficial; it's essential for maintaining harmony between your goals and your ever-evolving life circumstances. This approach ensures that your strategies remain as adaptive and resilient as possible, enabling you to meet changing demands with confidence and ease.

Importance of Review and Adaptation

Regularly reviewing and adapting your time management strategies is crucial, much like updating a map in real time as the terrain changes. This process helps you stay aligned with your current needs and goals, which can vary significantly over time due to changes in your personal and professional life and shifts in your ADHD symptoms. For instance, a strategy that worked well during a stable period may become ineffective during a more turbulent phase. By staying attuned to these changes and adjusting your methods accordingly, you can ensure that your strategies continue to support your productivity and well-being.

Methods for Effective Review

Conducting effective self-reviews involves several essential practices that can help you assess the suitability of your time management strategies. Periodic reflection sessions are vital. These can be scheduled monthly or quarterly and involve a thorough review of what's working and what isn't. During these sessions, ask yourself questions like, "Which strategies have improved my productivity?" and "What has been causing me stress?" This can help identify areas for improvement.

Additionally, feedback from trusted individuals such as colleagues, friends, or coaches who understand your challenges with ADHD can provide invaluable insights. They may observe patterns you overlook and suggest practical adjustments. Furthermore, maintaining journals or using digital apps to track your daily activities and productivity can provide concrete data on your progress and the effectiveness of different strategies. This ongoing record not only aids in self-reflection but also helps in fine-tuning your approach to time management.

Adaptation Strategies

Based on the outcomes of your reviews, adapting your time management strategies can take several forms. For instance, scaling certain practices up or down can better align with your current needs. If a tool or method has become less effective, modify it or replace it with something more suitable. For example, if you've relied on digital tools for scheduling but find them overwhelming, it might be time to switch to a more straightforward, tactile system like a physical planner.

Introducing new tools or techniques can also rejuvenate your approach to time management. Innovations in digital apps that cater specifically to ADHD needs are continually emerging, and staying open to trying new solutions can lead to discoveries that significantly enhance your productivity. On the other hand, if specific strategies or tools no longer serve your needs, it's okay to let them go. This trial, error, and refinement process is normal and necessary for finding what works for you.

Case Studies of Adaptation

Consider the experience of Ella, a project manager with ADHD, who found that her traditional method of using detailed daily to-do lists became overwhelming as her responsibilities increased. Through regular review, she realized that this method was no longer sustainable. By shifting to a weekly planning system with broader goals and fewer daily specifics, she was able to reduce her daily stress and focus more effectively on her priorities.

Another case is that of Lily, a freelance illustrator with ADHD, who initially used various apps to manage her projects and deadlines. Over time, she realized that juggling multiple apps was becoming a distraction. After a reflective review session, she decided to consolidate her task management into a single, comprehensive app that provided all the necessary functionalities. This change significantly streamlined her workflow, reducing cognitive load and allowing her to spend more time focused on her work.

TransThese adaptations highlight the importance of being flexible and responsive to your needs. By continuously evaluating and adjusting your strategies, you can maintain a time management system that copes with and thrives on the changes inherent in life with ADHD. Remember, these strategies aim not to achieve perfection but to foster an environment where you can perform at your best, adapting as you grow and as your circumstances evolve.

In wrapping up this chapter, the journey through adapting your time management strategies is a testament to the dynamic nature of living with ADHD. It's about making peace with perpetual change and using it as a catalyst for growth and improvement. As we transition into the next chapter, we'll explore how integrating these adaptive strategies into broader life contexts can further enhance your ability to manage time and achieve your goals.

10

TRANSFORMING YOUR LIFE AND MOTIVATIONAL INSIGHTS

TIME MANAGEMENT AS A TOOL FOR LIFE TRANSFORMATION

When you think of time management, you might picture planners,
calendars, and lists—a set of tools
to organize your day. But what if
we view time management as
something more profound, a transformative power that reshapes your
daily tasks and life? For those living
with ADHD, mastering time
management does more than help
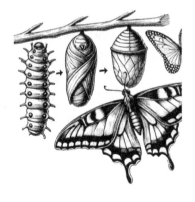
us remember appointments or meet deadlines; it becomes a
cornerstone for a more fulfilling, balanced, and prosperous
existence.

Understanding time management as a transformative process
opens up a world where each day is more than a series of tasks; it's

an opportunity to build the life you envision. Effective time management touches every aspect of life. It reduces stress by removing the chaos of unpredictability, which can be a significant source of anxiety, particularly for those with ADHD. With fewer surprises and less scrambling, your mental health finds a more stable foundation, free from the constant ups and downs that poor time management often brings.

Moreover, the benefits extend beyond your personal peace; they reach into your relationships. When you manage your time well, you're more present. Whether it's being punctual for a coffee date or being able to listen without distraction, the people in your life receive a more explicit message that they are valued. This reliability strengthens your relationships, building trust and understanding crucial for personal and professional growth.

On the professional front, imagine walking into your workplace with a clear plan for the day—understanding your priorities and having the time allocated to focus on what's important. This ability can drastically enhance your career success. Employers and colleagues start to see you as dependable and focused, qualities that can lead to greater responsibilities and opportunities. Your career trajectory can shift from one of missed opportunities and unfulfilled potential to one marked by achievements and advancements.

However, the most compelling aspect of viewing time management as a transformative tool is its role in realizing long-term aspirations. Each well-managed day is a stepping stone toward your larger life goals. Whether pursuing further education, building a business, or dedicating time to a passion project, managing your time directly affects your ability to make these dreams a reality. The sense of fulfillment and achievement that comes from reaching these milestones can be a powerful motivator, inspiring you to continue managing your time effectively.

Now, consider the stories of those who have embraced this expansive view of time and its management. There's the tale of a young writer named John who, once paralyzed by unmanaged deadlines and a chaotic schedule, started using strategic planning to carve out dedicated writing times throughout her week. This led to her first published novel and restored her belief in completing large, intimidating projects. Or the story of a father who struggled to balance work and family life, his time consumed by a demanding job and the chaos of ADHD. He enhanced his career by implementing rigorous time-blocking techniques and learning to prioritize tasks effectively. He reclaimed evenings and weekends with his family, deepening those relationships and creating a more harmonious home life.

These narratives are not just individual successes but invitations to view your daily struggles and triumphs through a broader lens. They illustrate how the disciplined application of time management strategies can alter life paths, turning everyday efforts into the foundation for more considerable successes.

As you reflect on these stories and insights, consider how effective time management principles might transform your life. Think about the areas where you feel unfulfilled or stressed and how better time management could bring peace and progress. Whether it's carving out time for health, relationships, career advancement, or personal growth, remember that each step you take in mastering your time is a step toward a more prosperous, more satisfying life, one well-managed moment at a time.

ESTABLISHING A PERSONAL TIME MANAGEMENT PHILOSOPHY

Navigating life with ADHD often means developing a unique approach to managing time that aligns closely with your personal values, strengths, and life goals. Crafting a personal time management philosophy isn't just about choosing the right tools or techniques; it's about integrating these strategies into the core of who you are, making them a fundamental part of your identity. This integration helps cultivate a sense of consistency and effectiveness in managing your time, ultimately making daily tasks feel more natural and less forced.

Let's explore how you can develop your time management philosophy. Begin by reflecting on what truly matters to you. What are your core values? What goals drive you? Understanding these can help you identify the time management practices that resonate most strongly with you. For instance, if creativity is a central value, your time management approach might include dedicated blocks for brainstorming and free exploration, ensuring these activities are preserved amid more routine tasks. Similarly, if relationships are meaningful to you, you should carve out time in your schedule for family and friends, making this a priority as any work commitment.

Integrating time management into your identity requires a mindset that views it as a key to living your best life. It's about seeing every well-planned day not as a series of tasks completed but as a step toward realizing your personal and professional aspirations. This perspective can transform how you view time management—from a chore or a challenge to an essential component of your success and well-being.

Successful individuals often operate under clear personal time management philosophies that guide their daily actions and decisions. Consider the philosophy of Scott a renowned academic who views time as a finite resource to be allocated as judiciously as financial investments. She prioritizes tasks based on deadlines and their potential to impact her long-term research goals and career growth. Another example is a tech entrepreneur who integrates mindfulness into his time management, ensuring that each segment of his day includes space for reflection, which he believes fuels innovation and creativity. These philosophies aren't just about getting through the day; they're about crafting a lifestyle that brings out their best selves.

However, developing a personal time management philosophy isn't a one-time event—it requires ongoing adjustment and refinement. Continually revisiting and refining your approach ensures it aligns with your evolving goals and life circumstances. Life is dynamic—your responsibilities might change, new goals might emerge, and what works today might not work tomorrow. Regularly assessing the effectiveness of your time management strategies in the context of your current life can help you make necessary adjustments, keeping your approach both practical and relevant.

This process of continual refinement goes beyond simply adjusting your schedule—it's a journey of deeper self-exploration. It's an opportunity to regularly connect with your core values and ensure that managing your time reflects who you are and aspire to be. This alignment is crucial because when your day-to-day actions are congruent with your deeper values and goals, managing your time becomes more fulfilling and less of a struggle.

In embedding these practices into your life, consider setting aside time each month or at the start of each new season to review your time management philosophy. Ask yourself whether your current practices serve you well, what challenges you face, and what goals require more focus. Use this insight to adjust your approach, experiment with new techniques, or abandon those that no longer serve you. This regular reflection ensures your time management strategies remain effective and deepens your understanding of yourself and your needs, enhancing your overall quality of life.

As you embark on this path, remember that your time management philosophy is a personal blueprint for how you navigate your days. When used wisely, it's a tool that can enhance your effectiveness, reduce your stress, and bring you closer to the life you envision for yourself. With each day managed according to a philosophy that reflects your values and goals, you're actively crafting a rich, fulfilling life aligned with your deepest aspirations.

THE FUTURE OF ADHD AND TIME MANAGEMENT: TRENDS AND TOOLS

As we look to the horizon, the future of managing ADHD in our fast-evolving world holds promise with the advent of groundbreaking technologies and insightful research. The potential for these advancements to significantly improve the lives of individuals with ADHD can inspire a sense of hope and optimism.

Artificial Intelligence (AI) is making significant inroads into personalized health and productivity tools. For those of us with ADHD, AI-driven planners and apps could soon predict our productive ebbs and flows, adapting our real-time schedules to align with our cognitive states. Imagine an app that learns from your behavior and can expect when you are most likely to be in a focused state. It could then schedule your most demanding tasks in these periods and suggest breaks or less cognitively demanding activities when your focus wanes. This kind of technology does more than manage time; it harmonizes our day-to-day tasks with our brain's natural rhythms, potentially reducing the stress of trying to fit our diverse neurological needs into a rigid schedule.

Virtual reality (VR) offers another intriguing frontier. VR technology can simulate office environments for task rehearsal, which could benefit job training and performance for people with ADHD. These simulations could help develop time management skills in a virtual setting that mimics real-life scenarios but without the real-world consequences of missing deadlines or forgetting appointments. This safe, controlled environment allows for practice and repetition, which can help solidify these skills before applying them in the workplace or daily routines.

The ongoing research into ADHD and time management is equally promising. Recent studies are beginning to shed light on the neurobiological fluctuations throughout the day in individuals with ADHD, offering more in-depth insights into why certain times may be better for cognitive tasks. This research could lead to more personalized time management strategies based on a scientific understanding of ADHD physiology rather than a one-size-fits-all approach. As our knowledge deepens, so will the tools and techniques at our disposal, ensuring they are scientifically grounded and highly tailored to our unique needs.

Predictions for the future of ADHD management suggest a greater integration of technology in both personal and professional spheres. As workplaces become more understanding and accommodating of neurodiversity, we might see wider adoption of tools designed to enhance productivity for individuals with ADHD. Furthermore, lifestyle trends are likely to continue evolving toward more flexible work environments—such as remote work and flexible hours—which can be highly beneficial for managing ADHD. These trends accommodate and celebrate different ways of thinking and managing time, potentially leading to more innovative and inclusive work cultures.

Preparing for these future trends and technologies involves staying informed and adaptable. It's essential to keep abreast of new tools and research, actively seeking to understand how they can be integrated into your life. Experimentation is critical—what works for one person might not work for another, so trying out new methods and tools to find what best suits your specific needs is essential. Building a support network with professionals who can provide insights and guidance on new developments can help you navigate these changes effectively.

As these advancements unfold, the potential for significantly improved quality of life for those of us with ADHD is immense. By embracing new technologies, staying informed about research, and preparing to adapt to evolving trends, you can ensure that your strategies for managing time and ADHD are as dynamic and resilient as the world around you. This proactive approach not only keeps you at the forefront of ADHD management but also empowers you to take full advantage of emerging opportunities to enhance your productivity and well-being.

EMPOWERING YOURSELF FOR ONGOING SUCCESS IN TIME MANAGEMENT

Empowering yourself in managing ADHD isn't just about finding the right tools—it's about fully integrating time management into your daily life. This empowerment comes from within through self-reflection, self-education, and self-advocacy. These methods do more

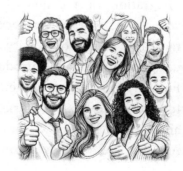

than help you manage your sched-
ule; they help you understand and navigate your needs, turning
what might be perceived as weaknesses into well-managed
strengths.

Self-reflection is a powerful tool, especially when tailored to
understanding how ADHD affects your time management.
Regularly reflecting on your day or week can provide crucial
insights into what strategies are working and what areas need
adjustment. This could be as simple as spending a few minutes
each evening reviewing what tasks were completed and how you
felt about your productivity. Such moments of reflection help you
stay aligned with your goals and foster a more in-depth understanding of how your unique brain operates, which is critical for
adapting time management strategies to fit your needs.

Self-education about ADHD and time management is also vital. It
involves staying informed about the latest research and strategies
to help you cope with ADHD symptoms. This might mean reading
books, attending workshops, or participating in webinars dedicated to ADHD management. Knowledge is power, and the more
you understand how ADHD affects time perception and task
execution, the better equipped you are to create effective management strategies. Moreover, understanding the scientific and
psychological facets of ADHD can also aid in self-advocacy,
providing you with the necessary tools to communicate your
needs and challenges to others, whether in personal relationships
or professional settings.

Self-advocacy is more than just asking for accommodations or
explaining your challenges; it's about asserting your needs and
ensuring that the surrounding structures support your success.
This could involve negotiating deadlines, presenting your work
methods to colleagues, or setting boundaries with family and

friends regarding your time and commitments. Effective self-advocacy ensures that your environment is conducive to your success, respecting and accommodating your unique way of interacting with the world.

Leveraging community resources plays a crucial role in sustaining success in time management. Communities, whether online or in person, provide a wealth of resources—workshops, seminars, and courses that offer both learning and support. These resources are invaluable for continual improvement and adaptation of time management strategies. They provide education and a sense of belonging and understanding, which can be incredibly empowering. For instance, participating in an ADHD support group workshop might introduce you to new time management tools or strategies you hadn't considered before, enriching your approach.

Maintaining motivation and momentum requires setting evolving challenges that keep you engaged and focused. This might mean setting increasingly complex goals as you master basic time management skills or finding new areas where improved time management could significantly impact you. Connecting with mentors or coaches who understand ADHD can also provide a source of motivation and accountability, helping you stay committed to your time management goals over the long term.

Celebrating personal growth is essential. Recognizing and honoring the milestones in your time management journey reinforces the positive impacts of your efforts. Celebrations can be simple, such as taking a moment to acknowledge a week of successful planning or, more significantly, treating yourself to a weekend getaway after completing a major project. These celebrations provide well-deserved recognition and reinforce the habits and strategies that led to your successes, encouraging their continued use.

In weaving these strategies into the fabric of your life, you transform time management from a daily challenge into a personal strength. This transformation is not just about getting through the day or managing tasks—it's about building a framework for living that honors your unique needs and harnesses your strengths. Through self-empowerment, community support, and ongoing celebration of your achievements, you create a sustainable approach to managing time that supports your productivity and overall happiness and well-being.

As this chapter concludes, remember that each strategy discussed here is more than just a way to manage time—it's a step toward a more empowered, fulfilled, and balanced life. Whether through self-reflection, education, advocacy, or community engagement, these techniques provide the tools to transform your relationship with time. They offer more than just productivity improvements; they provide a pathway for personal growth and success tailored to the unique rhythms of living with ADHD.

TAKE YOUR JOURNEY TO THE NEXT LEVEL!

Download your Bonus Companion Worksheets and Resources Workbook by simply scanning the QR code or visit the link below. We willsend you a PDF copy instantly.

www.adhdworkbookdownload.com

This workbook includes everything referenced in the book—worksheets, apps, best practices, and even more additional tools to help you succeed.

Don't stop here—keep striving for improvement!

"If you are not scared of your dreams then your dreams are not big enough."

— ALBERT EINSTEIN

CONCLUSION

As we conclude this guide, let's pause to acknowledge the significant role you've played in this journey. From unraveling the intricate relationship between ADHD and time management to exploring a multitude of strategies to boost focus and productivity, this book has been a testament to your 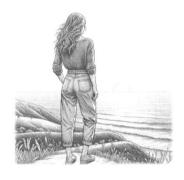 empowerment and hope. We've delved into how ADHD influences our perception of time, discussed ways to tailor tools and techniques for managing daily tasks, and stressed the importance of lifestyle adjustments that bolster your overall well-being. Together, we've navigated the complexities of communication, collaboration, and the essential adaptation of traditional time management methods to better suit the ADHD mind.

The core message we've revisited throughout is one of profound empowerment—recognizing that you, as an individual with

ADHD, can master time management and lead a productive, less stressful life. The strategies and insights shared here are guidelines and tools for transformation, designed to be adapted and molded to fit your unique life tapestry.

Remember, the effectiveness of any time management strategy is deeply personal. What works wonderfully for one person might require adjustments for another. I encourage you to embrace personalization in every approach, tuning into your specific needs, habits, and preferences. It's about crafting a system that resonates with your lifestyle and supports your goals, putting you in the driver's seat of your time management journey.

I urge you to keep the spirit of experimentation alive. Be open to trying new techniques, tweaking existing ones, and being flexible as your circumstances evolve. Time management with ADHD is not static but dynamic, growing and adapting as you do.

A crucial aspect of this process is developing self-awareness and practicing self-compassion. Understand your patterns, recognize your strengths, and be kind to yourself through the ups and downs. Managing time with ADHD is not about achieving perfection but making progress that enhances your quality of life and brings you joy.

Now, I call on you to take the first step on this path if you haven't already. Whether implementing just one new strategy from this book, revisiting your personal and professional goals, or initiating a conversation about ADHD and time management with someone in your circle, begin where you feel most compelled.

As you progress, I encourage you to share your stories and successes. Your experiences can light the way for others and strengthen the sense of community and support vital for all of us navigating ADHD. Each shared story is a beacon of hope and a testament to the power of dedicated effort and personalized strategy. Remember, you are not alone on this journey. Together, we can overcome the challenges and celebrate the victories.

Thank you for sharing this part of your journey with me. Your courage, determination, and optimism are inspiring. May the strategies and insights from this book serve as valuable companions as you continue to navigate your unique path. Here's to mastering the art of time management together, each step an achievement, every day a new possibility. Celebrate your progress, no matter how small, for each step is a testament to your strength and resilience.

Finally, let me reassure you that while this journey may present challenges, the rewards of gaining greater control over your time and tasks are immeasurable. The path to mastering time management with ADHD is a journey worth embarking upon, filled with opportunities for growth, learning, and profound satisfaction. Embrace the journey, for it is not just about managing time but about discovering your potential and learning about yourself.

KEEPING THE GAME ALIVE

Now you have everything you need to master your time, it's time to pass on your newfound knowledge and show other readers where they can find the same help.

Simply by leaving your honest opinion of this book on Amazon, you'll show other adults with ADHD where they can find the information they're looking for, and push their passion for time management forward.

Thank you for your help. The topic of time management is kept alive when we pass on our knowledge – and you're helping me to do just that.

Simply scan the QR code or visit the link below to leave your review on Amazon:

www.adhdtimemgmtreview.com

REFERENCES

1 ADDitude. (n.d.). *Time management skills for ADHD brains: Practical advice.* https://www.additudemag.com/time-management-skills-adhd-brain/

2 Fayyazi Bordbar, M. R., Zare, H., & Farhangnia, P. (2019). *Comparison of quality of life, productivity, functioning, and satisfaction in adults with ADHD and the general population. Journal of Attention Disorders, 24*(14), 2068–2079. https://www.ncbi.nlm.nih.gov/pmc/articles/PMC6935829/

3 Murnan, J. (2023, February 10). *The 11 best ADHD apps.* Healthline. https://www.healthline.com/health/adhd/top-iphone-android-apps

4 ADDitude. (n.d.). *15 apps, tools, and gadgets for ADHD brains.* https://www.additudemag.com/adhd-productivity-apps-tools/

5 Morin, A. (2023, August 15). *How to use a planner for ADHD.* Verywell Mind. https://www.verywellmind.com/adhd-friendly-daily-planner-tips-20902

6 ADDitude. (n.d.). *Born this way: Personal stories of life with ADHD.* https://www.additudemag.com/adhd-personal-stories-real-life-people-living-with-adhd/

7 Coombes, A. (2022, April 28). *3 to-do list apps that actually work with ADHD.* Zapier. https://zapier.com/blog/adhd-to-do-list/

8 ADDitude. (n.d.). *Easily distracted? 9 productivity tricks for ADHD minds.* https://www.additudemag.com/slideshows/easily-distracted-9-productivity-tricks-for-adhd-minds/

9 ADDitude. (n.d.). *ADHD and anxiety: Understanding the link & how to cope.* https://www.additudemag.com/adhd-and-anxiety-symptoms-coping/

10 ADDitude. (n.d.). *ADHD apps: Time management and productivity tools.* https://www.additudemag.com/adhd-apps-tools-time-management-productivity/

11 Focumon. (2022, November 17). *The power of gamification in task management.* https://www.focumon.com/blog/11-the-power-of-gamification-in-task-management

12 Mindomo. (2023, June 22). *Unlocking the power of ADHD mind maps: A complete guide.* https://www.mindomo.com/blog/adhd-mind-map/

13 Parnes, M. (2023, March 14). *How to wind the Pomodoro technique for ADHD.* Psych Central. https://psychcentral.com/adhd/how-to-adapt-the-pomodoro-technique-adhd

14 Stoddard, A. (2023, May 16). *Manage your ADHD emotions.* WebMD. https://www.webmd.com/add-adhd/emotion-stress

15 Architectural Digest. (2023, July 25). *How to design an ADHD-friendly home.*

https://www.architecturaldigest.com/reviews/home-improvement/design-an-adhd-friendly-home

16 Molitor, J. (2023, October 25). *ADHD and effective motivation strategies.* Psychology Today. https://www.psychologytoday.com/us/blog/on-your-way-with-adhd/202310/adhd-and-effective-motivation-strategies

17 Psych Central. (2023, April 22). *Meeting your goals when you have ADHD: 9 helpful tips.* https://psychcentral.com/adhd/meeting-your-goals-when-you-have-adhd

18 ClickUp. (2024). *10 best ADHD productivity software tools & apps 2024.* https://clickup.com/blog/adhd-productivity-tools/

19 Smith, M., & Segal, J. (2023, January 23). *Tips for managing adult ADHD.* HelpGuide. https://www.helpguide.org/articles/add-adhd/managing-adult-adhd-attention-deficit-disorder.htm

20 Healthline. (2023, August 19). *How to maintain your focus with ADHD.* https://www.healthline.com/health/mental-health/adhd-quick-focus-boosts

21 WebMD. (2023, July 9). *ADHD diet and nutrition: Foods to eat & foods to avoid.* https://www.webmd.com/add-adhd/adhd-diets

22 ADDitude. (n.d.). *Best fitness advice for adults with ADHD.* https://www.additudemag.com/exercise-fitness-tips-adult-adhd/

23 ADDitude. (n.d.). *How to get organized with adult ADHD.* https://www.additudemag.com/how-to-get-organized-with-adhd/

24 The ADHD Minimalist. (2023, March 5). *How minimalism can reduce ADHD symptoms.* https://theadhdminimalist.com/how-minimalism-can-reduce-adhd-symptoms/

25 Goblinx ADHD. (2023, September 19). *Effective communication strategies for ADHD employees.* https://www.goblinxadhd.com/blog/effective-communication-strategies-for-adhd-employ/

26 ADDitude. (n.d.). *How to delegate with an ADHD brain.* https://www.additudemag.com/how-to-delegate-with-adhd/

27 ADDitude. (n.d.). *Sensitive to criticism? How to respond gracefully.* https://www.additudemag.com/sensitive-to-criticism-how-to-respond-gracefully/#:~

28 Healthline. (2023, July 14). *ADHD and empathy: What's the link?.* https://www.healthline.com/health/adhd/adhd-and-empathy

29 CareClinic. (2023, August 11). *Bullet journal for ADHD: Organize your thoughts.* https://careclinic.io/bulletjournal-adhd/

30 Sachs Center. (2023, March 20). *Time management challenges with ADHD: Time optimism.* https://sachscenter.com/time-management-challenges-with-adhd-time-optimism/

31 Great Careers. (2023, June 5). *Living with ADHD and ADHD-friendly tools for success.* https://greatcareers.org/living-with-adhd-and-friendly-tools-for-success/

32 TimeCamp. (2023, May 17). *ADHD time management - Get things done.* https://www.timecamp.com/blog/adhd-time-management/

33 ADDitude. (n.d.). *Famous people with ADHD: Simone Biles, Emma Watson.* https://www.additudemag.com/slideshows/famous-people-with-adhd/

34 ADDitude. (n.d.). *Emotional resilience with ADHD: Coping with challenges.* https://www.additudemag.com/emotional-resilience-adhd-coping/

35 Psych Breakthrough. (2023, July 3). *How tech innovations are transforming adult ADHD care.* https://www.psychbreakthrough.com/breakthrough-blog/beyond-the-debate-how-tech-innovations-are-transforming-adult-adhd-care

Made in United States
Orlando, FL
26 May 2025

61614971R00089